NURSING ROBOTS
*Robotic Technology and
Human Caring for the Elderly*

SUPERVISING EDITORS
Tetsuya Tanioka
Yuko Yasuhara
Kyoko Osaka
Hirokazu Ito
Rozzano Locsin

FUKURO SHUPPAN Publishing
ふくろう出版

Nursing Robots

Robotic Technology and Human Caring for the Elderly

Published on 25, March 2017

The Authors: Tetsuya Tanioka and Associates

The Publisher: FUKURO Publishing
1-23, Takayanagi-Nishimachi, Kita Ward, Okayama City, Okayama
Prefecture, Japan, 700-0035
http://www.296.jp   e-mail: info@296.jp
Phone: 81-86-255-2181   Facsimile: 81-86-255-6324

ISBN978-4-86186-689-0 C3047

Copyright (C) Tetsuya Tanioka and Associates, 2017.
All Rights Reserved. No part of this book may be reproduced or utilized in
any form electronic or mechanical, including photocopying, reprinting, or on
any information storage or retrieval system, without permission in writing
from the publisher.

Printed in Japan.

FOREWORD

As I began reading a draft of this book, *Nursing Robots: Robotic Technology and Human Caring for the Elderly,* by Tanioka, Locsin and colleagues and feeling the excitement of new opportunities for nursing, I recalled a much earlier nursing publication that generated a similar sense of excitement. That was an article in *Nursing Outlook* titled "Patients' Work in the Technologized Hospital", by Strauss, Fagerhaugh, Suczek and Wiener (1981). The specific stimulus in this new book that triggered my memory was the discussion about what constitutes the work of nursing. In the "Patients' Work" article, specific activities (mental, social, physical) required of patients so they could benefit from their hospital stay were linked to the demands for nursing care from the perspective of Orem's Self-Care Deficit Nursing Theory.

So now we have 21st century and even 22nd century thinking in nursing! And again, or should I say, still, thinking in nursing is usefully and appropriately guided by explicit general and middle-range theories of nursing, based on an integrated philosophical framework conveying a developed nursing perspective.

I am reminded too of a workshop Locsin and I facilitated with deans of nursing education programs in the Philippines some years ago, in particular, Locsin's image of "sacred cows". The workshop was focused on a revolution in the nursing curriculum, and Locsin's point was that sacred cows had to be recognized as such before the doorway would open to a truly revolutionary curriculum design. The same may be said of the aim of revolutionizing the work of nurses and nursing in hospitals and elder care institutions. We like to say in nursing – and I have no doubt said it myself – that the nurse can never be taken out of nursing. Tanioka, Locsin and their colleagues have shown us in this work the truth of that statement – but with new meaning. In the not-too-distant future, "nurses" may actually be what they term Humanoid Robot Nurses (HRNs). As bizarre and perhaps even off-putting as this prediction may seem to many of us, this book helps us see how the idea of caring as central to Nursing can expand our understanding and get us pass the initial impulse

i

Foreword

to reject a future that seamlessly integrates personified anthropomorphic machine technologies as partners in care.

Serendipitously, just the day before I began reading the draft manuscript of this new book, I had seen the movie *Hidden Figures*. I was struck from the very beginning of that film by the use of the word "computers". When I heard it, I thought immediately of "machines in boxes", room-size at first and later palm-size and smaller. But what the term referred to in the movie was persons – the persons who solved the mathematical problems that held the secret of putting humans into space. The computers in that movie were persons! And now Tanioka, Locsin and their colleagues are describing very real possibilities that computers (machines in boxes) will become humanoid and perhaps even human.

As I was reading, I wondered about growing in caring. Just as humans express emotions and realize caring intentions, and grow from those experiences, Tanioka and Locsin in Chapter 14 propose that nurse-humanoids will grow in their ability to truly understand and communicate caring in meaningful, relevant ways in nursing situations with elders and in hospital settings. Their proposal suggests that personhood (living grounded in caring) is not out of the question in the future for HRNs.

Alan Barnard, in Chapter 10, notes that "Responsibility for the future of nursing practice and healthcare must involve more than robots doing nursing work, and acceptance of change is a logical aspiration. The degree of adaptation necessary in order for nurses to maintain person-focused care and participate as leaders will be enormous, and the implications even bigger". Barnard's challenge is acknowledged and addressed in most of the chapters in the book.

In the closing chapter, Tanioka and Locsin repeat the key question guiding their work: "What is required of humanoid robots in order to establish a trusting relationship between them and human persons?" Answering this question will require a new multi-dimensional consideration of what it means to be human in every realm, including but not limited to the theological, sociocultural, and physico-physiological dimensions. Relational questions need to be explored directly.

Foreword

For example, the issue of the healthcare robot as servant versus partner calls for the consideration of mutuality in light of different capabilities, differences that in 20th century thinking were organized as a hierarchy.

Finally, on a personal note, I am awed and humbled to see how the nursing theory that Anne Boykin and I developed in the early 1980's, the theory of Nursing As Caring, is recognized as such a relevant and fertile field for thinking about the human issues surrounding health-caring robots for nursing and healthcare in the 21st century and beyond. I am grateful to Tetsuya Tanioka, Rozzano C. Locsin, and their colleagues for sharing a type of thinking that can move caring practice into the future, with the vehicle being nurses and other humans as we know them today, accompanied by HRNs and other humanoid healthcare workers.

Reference

Strauss AL, Fagerhaugh S, Suczek B, Wiener C: Patients' work in the technologized hospital. Nursing Outlook, Vol. 29, No. 7, pp. 404-412, 1981.

Savina Schoenhofer, RN, PhD

Board member,

Anne Boykin Institute for the Advancement of Caring in Nursing

Florida Atlantic University

Christine E. Lynn College of Nursing

Boca Raton, FL 33431

USA

iii

Preface

If we do not find a workable solution to the problems of a low birth rate and longevity, Japanese society will face a critical shortage in the labor force caused by a dwindling working population, in contrast to an increasing number of aging people. This book provides us the opportunity to open our eyes to the future, and to consider some solutions. Introducing robot technology to the medical and welfare fields, to the social environment, and most importantly, to the nursing practice settings are laudable ways to try to come up with actual pracicable solutions. The Japanese government has provided a New Robot Strategy beginning in 2015 [1-3]. Advances in technology enabled the rapid development of humanoid robots, which were designed for use in companies, department stores [4], hospitals, and geriatric health service facilities. Today, in the face of these same conditions, more sophisticated robots are now being constructed, which include "watch-over" robots and communication robots that are currently in development [5, 6].

Nevertheless, contemporary technological advancements necessitate serious reflection on this central question: "Is it possible to develop robots to replace humans and resolve the issues of shortage of care givers?" Even if these robots can be developed for actual use, the kind of functions and ethical attitudes undergirding their artificial moral agency (AMA) should be addressed and geared toward caring for older adults, especially those with dementia.

This book, Nursing Robots: Robotic Technology and Human Caring for the Elderly, sets itself apart with its own heft and magnitude, considering that the theme explored here requires a much broader perspective than those taken by researchers in a specific field. Discussion of this grand challenge from a more interdisciplinary viewpoint entails the consideration of robotics, science, technology, nursing, and engineering, where they all come together as an amalgamation of disciplinary foci that engages one practical concern: caring for elderly patients in a future of technological advancements.

Preface

The main idea of the book arose from Dr. Tetsuya Tanioka's vision of the ultimate technological marvel that would surface in the years to come. An author and principal editorial supervisor of this book, he once questioned the status quo of the social policy on people with physical disability and their rehabilitative treatments and activities. He based his arguments from his long clinical career of psychiatric nursing that started in 1988. He was sympathetic to the normalization principle [7-9], which is the current basis of his ways of thinking towards practices and research in clinical situations. He wanted to prevent patients with schizophrenia from succumbing to the drug-induced Parkinsonism effects caused by antipsychotic drugs. In order to do this, he thought it necessary to clarify human movement from the viewpoint of engineering because patients with Parkinsonism showed ambulation activity specific to this disease. In this way, he started to focus on the research based on the engineering of human movements. While researching at the Graduate School of Engineering of the Kochi University of Technology, he devoted himself to interdisciplinary research in collaboration with the Kochi Medical School researchers, through which he obtained his PhD in 2002, coming out with his study "A Sensor-based System for Rehabilitating the Gait of Persons with Parkinsonism: Assessment, Programming and Implementation" [10, 11]. This was awarded two patents. Using this case to start, he gradually formed his base to develop an interdisciplinary nursing research team with the inclusion of viewpoints from engineering.

He continued his research and came to be influenced by two distinguished researchers, Drs. Rozzano C. Locsin and Fuji Ren.

Dr. Tanioka met Dr. Locsin in 2005. Dr. Locsin came to Japan along with a delegation from Florida Atlantic University where he worked. He made an academic agreement with the Faculty of Medicine of the Department of Nursing of Tokushima University. It was at a dinner celebration that Dr. Tanioka met Dr. Locsin and hit it off with him as they discussed the state of the research in nursing, caring, and technology. Dr. Locsin's own book, "Technological Competency as Caring in Nursing," became a major influence in Dr. Tanioka's research investigations. Dr.

v

Preface

Tanioka translated this book into the Japanese language. It is now in its third printing.

Dr. Locsin is a nurse and nursing theorist who described the possible coexistence between technology and caring in nursing, extending such coexistence to the harmonious integration of technology and caring in nursing [12, 13] and this time, even though Dr. Tanioka took an interest in Dr. Locsin's theory, it took some time for him to understand it thoroughly, due to the many definitions of the term *technology* in the context of its ontology and epistemological value. In addition, he thought that Dr. Locsin's ideas, based on the so-called "posthuman", came too early in the decade and may perhaps only be more meaningful in the distant future.

In 2005, Drs. Tanioka and Locsin started collaborative research [14]. Through discussions as partners, their trusting relationship was established in their co-authored research studies and presentations in international conferences. Twelve years have passed since they first met, and now Dr. Tanioka has come to think of Dr. Locsin's theories as especially pertinent, and applicable in all levels of human caring relationships and in all settings. Looking at the relationship between current technology and nursing issues, ethical considerations, and humanoid nursing robots of the future, readers might say that Dr. Tanioka's current view is entirely appropriate.

Drs. Tanioka and Ren assumed their posts at Tokushima University at the same time in 2002. They met at a seminar of the university faculty development office, and found that they both aimed at analyzing human emotions. It was natural that they soon engaged themselves in launching their new collaborative research importing this allied issue to human care. Their collaborative research opened a new avenue for further study. This led Dr. Tanioka to find a way to measure human emotions. Dr. Ren was a leading researcher of the information processing and the natural language processing (NLP) projects. He was a proponent of the Mental State Transition Network Model [15], as well. He studied humanoid robots using NLP, speech recognition, and image processing. In their collaborative research, they estimated human emotional changes using electroencephalographic activities, in

vi

order to analyze human empathic understanding required for human nurses [16].

Dr. Tanioka was granted a research promotion for robot development from leading Japanese enterprises in 2007. He launched a new research project on "humanoid robots" to clarify human nurses' roles in human caring. Concurrently, the Ministry of Economy, Trade and Industry and the Ministry of Health and Welfare in Japan started promoting the introduction of devices in nursing care and practice to reduce the costs of nursing. The study posited the introduction of care robots into the medical field, and discussed their part in monitoring details of the work of nurses and care workers who worked for elderly persons in hospitals and institutions, as well as the mutual relationship between patient and nurse, and the relationship among patient, nurse, and robot [17-27]. In 2013, the support program was launched based on the policy of the Japanese government [28].

Organization of the book

This book is divided into chapters which were clustered according to the themes of the three major parts.

PART 1 (Chapters 1 through 4) describes the thoughtful and serious concerns about the rapidly aging population, very low birth rate, and current developmental state of rehabilitation/support robots for the elderly in Japan, and the objective evaluation methods of care for the elderly with dementia.

PART 2 (Chapters 5 through 9) describes the communication capabilities required for humanoid nursing robots, and for the future of robot care in 2050.

PART 3 (Chapters 10 through 14) describes the possibility of relating in nursing, technologies in healthcare, caring, humanoid nurse robots, artificial intelligence, and corresponding health issues. Also, in the Chapter 11, Dr. Tanioka's The Transactive Relationship Theory of Nursing (TRETON): A Model for Nursing Engagement of Healthcare Robots and Human Persons [29] has been posted. Moreover, Chapters 11 and 14 are the core content of this book.

Drs. Carl Benedikt Frey and Michael A. Osborn predict that intellectual works will be replaced by computers with sense [30]. Could complicated judgments in the

Preface

field of nursing really be performed by humanoid robots and artificial intelligence? If so, how should we nurses change our work style following the introduction of humanoid nursing robots? This book will examine the past researches by the authors as well as the possibility of cooperation between human nurses and humanoid nursing robots, seen in the context of the aging Japanese society.

Yuko Yasuhara

Kyoko Osaka

Hirokazu Ito

References

[1] Robotic Care Devices Portal: Robotic Devices for Nursing Care Project. Portalhttp://robotcare.jp/?lang=en (Accessed 10 November 2016)

[2] Ministry of Economy, Trade and Industry: Joint Press Release with the Ministry of Health, Labour and Welfare, Revision of the Four Priority Areas to Which Robot Technology is to be introduced in Nursing Care of the Elderly — Three priority items have been newly designated, including bathing.
http://www.meti.go.jp/english/press/2014/0203_02.html
(Accessed 10 November 2016)

[3] Nursing Care and Robots: Ministry of Economy, Trade and Industry, Respond to actual needs with technology!
http://www.meti.go.jp/english/publications/pdf/journal2013_04.pdf
(Accessed 10 November 2016)

[4] Humanoid robot starts work at Japanese department store: TECHNOLOGY NEWS, Apr 20, 2015.
http://www.reuters.com/article/us-japan-robot-store-idUSKBN0NB1OZ20150420

[5] Nishiura Y, Inoue T, Nihei M: Appropriate talking pattern of an information support robot for people living with dementia: A case study. Journal of Assistive Technologies, Vol.8, No.4, pp. 177-187, 2013.

[6] Wada K, Shibata T, Saito T, Tanie K: Effects of robot-assisted activity for elderly

people and nurses at a day service center. Proceedings of the IEEE, Vol. 92, No. 11, pp.1780-1788, 2004.

DOI: 10.1109/JPROC.2004.835378

[7] Nirje B: The normalization principle and its human management implications. In Kugel R & Wolfensberger W (Eds.), Changing patterns in residential services for the mentally retarded. Washington, D.C.: President's Committee on Mental Retardation, 1969.

[8] Wolfensberger W: The Principle of Normalization in Human Services Toronto, Canada: National Institute on Mental Retardation, 1972.

[9] Nirje B: The basis and logic of the normalization principle. Australian and New Zealand Journal of Developmental Disabilities, Vol. 11, No. 2, pp. 65-68, 1985.

[10] Kai Y, Tanioka T, Inoue Y, Matsuda T, Sugawara K, Takasaka Y, Nagamine I: A walking support/evaluation machine for patients with parkinsonism, The Journal of Medical Investigation, Vol. 51, No. 1-2, pp.117-124, 2004.

[11] Tanioka T, Kai Y, Matsuda T, Inoue Y, Sugawara K, Takasaka Y, Tsubahara A, Matsushita Y, Nagamine I, Tada T, Hashimoto F: Real-time measurement of frozen gait in patient with parkinsonism using a sensor-controlled walker. The Journal of Medical Investigation, Vol.51, No.1-2, pp. 108-116, 2004.

[12] Locsin RC (Ed): Advancing Technology, Caring, and Nursing. Connecticut: Auburn House, Greenwood Publishing Group, Inc., 2001.

[13] Locsin RC (Ed): Technological competency as caring in nursing: A model for practice. Sigma Theta Tau International Press, Indianapolis, IN, 2005.

[14] Locsin RC, Tanioka T, Campling A: In Barnard A, Locsin RC, (Eds), Robots and Nursing Systems: Concepts, Relationships, and Practice. Technology and Nursing: Practice, Concepts and Issues.
Palgrave-Macmillan Co., Ltd., UK, 2006.

[15] Ren F, Dianbing J, Hua X, Kuroiwa S, Tanioka T, Zhong Z, Chengqing Z: Mental State Transition Network and Psychological Experiments. Proceedings of the Ninth IASTED International Conference on Artificial Intelligence and Soft Computing, Vol. 2005, No. 1, pp. 439-444, Benidorm, Sep. 2005.

Preface

[16] Osaka K, Chiba S, Tanioka T, Kawanishi C, Nagamine I, Ren F, Kuroiwa S, Tada T, Yamashita R, Kishimoto M, Nishimura M, Yamamoto A, Locsin RC, Takasaka Y: Estimating Emotion Changes Using Electroencephalographic Activities and its Clinical Application. Proceedings of 2005 IEEE International Conference on Natural Language Processing and Knowledge Engineering (IEEE NLP-KE'05), pp.830-834, Wuhan, China, Oct. 2005.

[17] Nagai Y, Tanioka T, Fuji S, Yasuhara Y, Sakamaki S, Taoka N, Locsin RC, Ren F, Matsumoto K: Needs and challenges of care robots in nursing care setting: A literature review. IEEE International Conference on Natural Language Processing and Knowledge Engineering (IEEE NLP-KE'10), pp. 292-295, Beijing, China, 2010.

[18] Fuji S, Date M, Nagai Y, Yasuhara Y, Tanioka T, Ren F: Research on the possibility of humanoid robots to assist in medical activities in nursing homes and convalescent wards. 2011 7th International Conference on Natural Language Processing and Knowledge Engineering (NLP-KE'11), pp. 459-463, Tokushima, Japan, 2011.

[19] Tanioka T, Locsin RC: Feasibility of developing nursing care robots. Proceeding of the 8th International Conference on Natural Language Processing and Knowledge, pp. 567-570, Hefei, China, 2012.

[20] Huang S, Tanioka T, Locsin RC, Parker M, Masory O: Functions of a caring robot in nursing. 2011 7th International Conference on Natural Language Processing and Knowledge Engineering (NLP-KE'11), pp. 425-429, Tokushima, Japan, 2011.

[21] Yasuhara Y, Tanioka T, Locsin RC: Adoption of medical welfare robots in medical environments and its ethical issues. Proceeding of the 8th International Conference on Natural Language Processing and Knowledge Engineering (KLP-KE '12), pp. 560-562, Hefei, China, 2012.

[22] Fuji S, Yasuhara Y, Tanioka T, Purnell MJ, Locsin RC: Required competencies for assistive-care robots for nursing. Proceeding of the 8th International Conference on Natural Language Processing and Knowledge Engineering (KLP-KE '12), pp. 557-559, Hefei, China, 2012.

Preface

[23] Fuji S, Ito H, Yasuhara Y, Shihong H, Tanioka T, Locsin RC: Discussion of Nursing Robot's Capability and Ethical Issues. Proceedings of the Sixth International Conference on Information (Info13), Tokyo, Japan, 2013.

[24] Osaka K, Tanioka T, Chiba S, et al.: Literature Study on Affective State Estimation for Human and Robot Interaction Using Physiological Indicators. INFORMATION, Vol.13, No.3, pp. 1099-1103, 2010.

[25] Yasuhara Y, Tamayama C, Kikukawa K, Osaka K, Tanioka T, Watanabe N, Chiba S, Miyoshi M, Locsin RC, Ren F, Fuji S, Ogasawara H, Mifune K: Required Function of the Caring Robot with Dialogue Ability for Patients with Dementia. AIA International Advanced Information Institute, Vol. 4, No. 1, pp. 31-42, 2012.

[26] Fuji S, Ito H, Yasuhara Y, Shihong H, Tanioka T, Locsin RC: Discussion of Nursing Robot's Capability and Ethical Issues. INFORMATION, Vol. 17, No. 1, pp. 349-354, 2014.

[27] Ito H, Miyagawa M, Kuwamura Y, Yasuhara Y, Tanioka T, Locsin RC: Professional Nurses' Attitudes towards the introduction of Humanoid Nursing Robots (HNRs) in Health Care Settings. Journal of Nursing and Health Sciences, pp. 73-81, 2015.

[28] Ministry of Economy, Trade and Industry Japan: priority areas in nursing care use of robot technology.
http://www.meti.go.jp/press/2013/02/20140203003/20140203003.html
(Accessed January 2016)

[29] Tanioka T: The Development of the Transactive Relationship Theory of Nursing (TRETON): A Nursing Engagement Model for persons and Robots and Humanoid Nursing Robots. Int J Nurs Clin Pract, Vol. 4, IJNCP-223, 2017.
DOI: 10.15344/2394-4978/2017/223

[30] Benedikt CF, Osborne MA: THE FUTURE OF EMPLOYMENT: HOW SUSCEPTIBLE ARE JOBS TO COMPUTERISATION? Sep. 17, 2013.
http://www.oxfordmartin.ox.ac.uk/downloads/academic/The_Future_of_Employment.pdf

xi

Prologue

If we do not find a workable solution to the problems of a low birth rate and longevity, Japanese society will face a critical shortage in the labor force caused by a dwindling working population, and an increasing number of aging citizens. Faced with these circumstances, the Japanese government devised a New Robot Strategy in 2015 [1-3]. Humanoid robot development was rapidly instituted – thanks to advancing technology – and designed to be used in companies, department stores [4], hospitals, and geriatric healthcare services and facilities. In addition, communication robots are being designed and developed as observation technologies [5, 6].

However, questions remain.

Is it possible to develop robots that would replace humans and thus resolve the issue of worker shortage, for example, in the healthcare profession? If such robots are developed and then come to exist, functional considerations and ethical attitudes will need critical appreciation if human society will insist on using them. For example, there is a need to ask ethico-moral questions such as "When caring for older adults, especially elderly persons with dementia, what functionalities should the robots have?" Addressing this concern needs a broader understanding of the consequences that may result from the utilization of robots in particular settings. Researchers in specific fields need to have a collaborative approach to decisions such as these, discussing the grand challenges from a more interdisciplinary viewpoint.

In the center of increasing research on robots in the fields of industries and business, Drs. Carl Benedikt Frey and Michael A. Osborn predicted that intellectual works will be replaced with computers with sense [7]. Could complicated judgments in the context of nursing really be performed by humanoid robots and artificial intelligence? Locsin (2017) [8] claims it can be done. Therefore, how should nurses change work styles following the introduction of humanoid nursing robots? In this book, past researches influencing human-to-human and human-to-robot

Prologue

relationships involving robot artificial super-intelligence are presented to aid in adopting appropriate technologies to meet the demands of future endeavors in healthcare. Cooperative undertakings with various interdisciplinary activities among human nurses and humanoid nursing robots will be a prospective visioning seen and realized from the perspective of Japanese human caring ideas for an aging society.

Tetsuya Tanioka
Rozzano C. Locsin

References

[1]   Robotic Care Devices Portal: Robotic Devices for Nursing Care Project. Portalhttp://robotcare.jp/?lang=en (Accessed 10 November 2016)

[2]   Ministry of Economy, Trade and Industry: Joint Press Release with the Ministry of Health, Labour and Welfare, Revision of the Four Priority Areas to Which Robot Technology is to be introduced in Nursing Care of the Elderly — Three priority items have been newly designated, including bathing —.
　http://www.meti.go.jp/english/press/2014/0203_02.html
　(Accessed 10 November 2016)

[3]   Nursing Care and Robots: Ministry of Economy, Trade and Industry, Respond to actual needs with technology!
　http://www.meti.go.jp/english/publications/pdf/journal2013_04.pdf
　(Accessed 10 November 2016)

[4]   REUTERS: Humanoid robot starts work at Japanese department store. TECHNOLOGY NEWS, 20 April 2015.
　http://www.reuters.com/article/us-japan-robot-store-idUSKBN0NB1OZ20150420

[5]   Nishiura Y, Inoue T, Nihei M: Appropriate talking pattern of an information support robot for people living with dementia: A case study. Journal of Assistive Technologies, Vol.8, No.4, pp. 177-187, 2013.

[6]   Wada K, Shibata T, Saito T, Tanie K: Effects of robot-assisted activity for elderly people and nurses at a day service center. Proceedings of the IEEE, Vol. 92, No. 11,

xiii

Prologue

pp.1780-1788, 2004. DOI: 10.1109/JPROC.2004.835378

[7] Frey CB, Osborne MA: The Future of Employment: How Susceptible Are Jobs to Computerisation? 17 September 2013.
http://www.oxfordmartin.ox.ac.uk/downloads/academic/The_Future_of_Employme nt.pdf

[8] Locsin RC: The Co-Existence of Technology and Caring in the Theory of Technological Competency as Caring in Nursing. Journal of Medical Investigation, Vol. 64, No. 1-2, pp. 160-164, 2017.

ACKNOWLEDGMENT

The editors express their gratitude to Fukurou Shuppan Publishing for publishing this visionary book on Nursing Robots. This work was partly supported by the Japan Society for the Promotion of Science (JSPS) KAKENHI Grant Number JP 24390477. Furthermore, the editors express their wholehearted gratitude to the contributors – experts in their own disciplines and professions of Nursing, Engineering, Computer Science, and Computer Engineering. Without their contributions this book *Nursing Robots: Robotic Technologies and Human Caring for the Elderly* would not be possible. Their commitment to sharing knowledge and their expertise are incomparable. They are visionaries who appreciate caring as an essential human attribute that is often considered the divide separating human beings and machines.

The editors thank Dr. Savina Schoenhofer who has perused the final drafts to ensure that the accurate and appropriate language is used in communicating the idea of human caring in nursing effectively and efficiently.

The editors thank Ms. Umehara and Ms. Bando, Dr. Tanioka's department secretaries for their tireless efforts to produce the best possible manuscript format and drafts.

And to all the visionaries now and in the future who share our vision of technologies and caring.

Thank you very much.

Tetsuya Tanioka, RN; PhD, FAAN
Yuko Yasuhara, RN; PhD
Kyoko Osaka, RN; PhD
Hirokazu Ito, RN; PhD
Rozzano C. Locsin, RN; PhD, FAAN
EDITORS

CONTENTS

FOREWORD (Savina Schoenhofer) _____ *i*

Preface _____ *iv*

Prologue _____ *xii*

ACKNOWLEDGMENT _____ *xv*

PART 01

The thoughtful and serious concerns about the rapidly aging population, very low birth rate, and current developmental state of rehabilitation/support robots for the elderly in Japan, and the objective evaluation of methods of care for the elderly with dementia.

Chapter I   Japan's Super-aging Society and Situational Concerns in
Providing a High Quality Human Care System ················· 2

By Mitsuko Omori

1. Introduction _____ *3*

2. Current status and future of Japan's aging population _____ *3*

3. Robotic solution in nursing care work _____ *6*

4. The environment surrounding the situation of medical treatment
and care of the elderly _____ *8*

5. Elderly health and welfare systems _____ *11*

6. Conclusion _____ *15*

Contents

Chapter II   Necessary Robotic Features to Support the Physical
Activities and Rehabilitation of the Elderly ····················· *19*

By Kazunori Yamazaki, Kenichi Sugawara,

Soichiro Koyama, Shigeo Tanabe

1. Introduction _____ *20*

2. Key development areas of personal care robots _____ *21*

3. ISO 13842 for the safety requirements for personal care robots _ *29*

4. Conclusion _____ *30*

Chapter III   Demand for Human Healthcare and Robotic Rehabilitation
Welfare Services among the Current Oldest and the Incoming
Elderly in Japanese Society ································· *35*

By Abbas Orand, Kotaro Takeda, Shigeo Tanabe

1. Introduction _____ *36*

2. Exercise assist robots _____ *36*

3. Independence assist robots _____ *40*

4. Care assist robots _____ *44*

5. Conclusion _____ *47*

Chapter IV   Evaluating the Effectiveness of Nursing Care Activities
for the Elderly with Dementia ······························· *51*

By Yuko Yasuhara, Shoko Fuji, Hiroko Sugimoto, Kaori Kato

1. Introduction _____ *52*

2. Method of objective evaluation _____ *53*

3. Intensive communication with elderly with dementia is effective in
maintaining their communication ability and daily life activity _ *56*

4. Can robots improve elderly persons' autonomic nervous system
and communication abilities? _____ *59*

xvii

Contents

5. Conclusion ⸺⸺⸺⸺⸺⸺⸺ *61*

PART 02

The communication capabilities required for humanoid nursing robots, and for the future of robot care in 2050.

Chapter V What are Robots? ···································· *68*
By Yoshihiro Kai

1. Introduction ⸺⸺⸺⸺⸺⸺⸺ *69*
2. The history of robots ⸺⸺⸺⸺⸺⸺ *69*
3. The definition of robots ⸺⸺⸺⸺⸺⸺ *70*
4. The basic components of robots ⸺⸺⸺⸺ *71*
5. The safety of robots ⸺⸺⸺⸺⸺⸺ *72*
6. Conclusion ⸺⸺⸺⸺⸺⸺⸺ *81*

Chapter VI Empathic Understanding in Human-Robot Communication: Influences on Caring in Nursing ············· *86*
By Kyoko Osaka

1. Introduction ⸺⸺⸺⸺⸺⸺⸺ *87*
2. Examination of prior study ⸺⸺⸺⸺⸺ *88*
3. Performance required in nursing robots ⸺⸺⸺ *89*
4. Conclusion ⸺⸺⸺⸺⸺⸺⸺ *101*

Chapter VII The Current State of Performance and Development of Natural Language Processing Required for Humanoid Caring Robots ·· *107*
By Kazuyuki Matsumoto

1. Introduction ⸺⸺⸺⸺⸺⸺⸺ *108*

xviii

Contents

2. Current stage of natural language processing for care robot – dialogue

system based on artificial intelligence techniques _____ *108*

3. Natural language understanding: Robust to unknown expressions *110*

4. Problems of implementation in a nursing care robot _____ *112*

5. Conclusion _____ *113*

ChapterⅧ Natural Language Processing Capabilities Required for

Humanoid Nursing Robots ·· *115*

By Fuji Ren, Kazuyuki Matsumoto

1. Introduction _____ *116*

2. Recognition of human emotions _____ *116*

3. Depression-tendency detection by emotion recognition _____ *117*

4. Prototype of humanoid robot _____ *119*

5. Conclusion _____ *121*

ChapterⅨ The Care Robot Trio "SHIN-GI-TAI" in 2050: Transactive

Relations among Psychiatrist, Patient, and Family ················· *123*

By Yueren Zhao, Tetsuya Tanioka, Rozzano C. Locsin,

Kyoko Osaka, Yuko Yasuhara

1. Introduction _____ *124*

2. Care robot trio "SHIN-GI-TAI" _____ *125*

3. The importance of healthcare practices based on caring partnership

among persons and healthcare robots _____ *127*

4. Rationalizing the influence of Buddhist thought in practice _ *128*

5. Issues concerning the Care Robot Trio "SHIN-GI-TAI" _____ *129*

6. Applications _____ *134*

7. Discussion _____ *140*

8. Conclusion _____ *144*

xix

Contents

PART 03

The possibility of relating in nursing, technologies in healthcare, caring, humanoid nurse robots, artificial intelligence, and corresponding health issues.

Chapter X A Critical Examination of Robotics and the Sacred in Nursing ·· *148*

By Alan Barnard

1. Introduction _____ *149*

2. Robots are the answer, but what was the question? _____ *150*

3. Nurses and robots _____ *152*

4. Robots and the sacred in nursing _____ *153*

5. Robots and the illusion of neutrality _____ *157*

6. Conclusion _____ *159*

Chapter XI The Transactive Relationship Theory of Nursing (TRETON): A Model for Nursing Engagement of Healthcare Robots and Human Persons ····························· *165*

By Tetsuya Tanioka

1. Introduction _____ *166*

2. Purpose _____ *168*

3. Artificial intelligence and healthcare robots features _____ *170*

4. Developing the Transactive Relationship Theory of Nursing (TRETON) _____ *171*

5. Theoretical assumptions _____ *172*

6. Evolving healthcare robots as intelligent machines _____ *174*

7. Enhancing nursing and caring in healthcare robots _____ *175*

8. The nursing encounter: Where all nursing occurs _____ *177*

9. Concerns about healthcare robots characteristics _____ *179*

xx

Contents

10. Performance of healthcare robots in a transactive relationship _ *180*

11. Healthcare robots and knowing in nursing *181*

12. Concluding statements emphasizing nursing practice applications _ *184*

ChapterXⅡ Artificiality of Intelligence in Human Caring Robots:
Ethical Issues for Nursing ·· *191*

By Hirokazu Ito, Yuko Yasuhara, Kyoko Osaka,

Tetsuya Tanioka, Rozzano C. Locsin

1. Introducing for nursing robot to medical environment *192*

2. Robots and human beings *194*

3. Research on contemporary ethical dilemmas of nurses and
engineers concerning humanoid nursing robots development and
utilization *196*

4. Ethical issues related to Artificial Intelligence (AI) *200*

5. Conclusion *203*

ChapterXⅢ The Relationship among Nursing, Technologies,
Caring, Humanoid Robots, and Artificial Intelligence ········· *207*

By Rozzano C. Locsin

1. Introduction *208*

2. Nursing practice and caring in nursing *208*

3. Consequences of nursing practice and intelligent machines __ *210*

4. Knowing persons as caring in nursing: A dynamic process of
nursing *211*

5. The future of nursing with persons and intelligent machines ___ *215*

6. Knowledge development through advancing nursing research *217*

7. Summary and conclusion *217*

8. Acknowledgment *219*

xxi

Contents

Chapter XIV Potential Developmental Issues in the Configuration of
"Nursing" in Humanoid Healthcare Robots ·················· *222*

By Tetsuya Tanioka, Rozzano C. Locsin

1. Introduction _____ *223*

2. Ethics and healthcare robots _____ *225*

3. Conclusion _____ *232*

Epilogue _____ *236*

Index _____ *243*

Endorsement _____ *251*

Biosketches of Authors _____ *254*

xxii

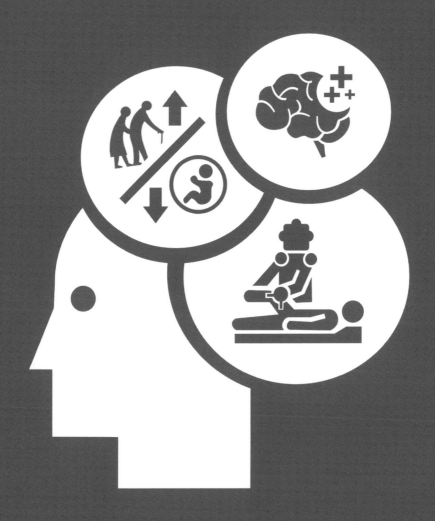

PART 01

The thoughtful and serious concerns about the rapidly aging population, very low birth rate, and current developmental state of rehabilitation/support robots for the elderly in Japan, and the objective evaluation of methods of care for the elderly with dementia.

© 2017 Illustrated by Leo Vicente Bollos

Part 1

> **Abstract**
>
> This chapter explains the current conditions of the aging society of Japan. The health of the elderly, health situations, and long-term care are described as challenges to healthcare. The health and welfare of the aging Japanese society makes it necessary to ensure their quality of life. Medical insurance and long-term care insurance are health systems that may require reforms. The Community-Based Integrated Care Systems (CBICS) is presented to meet the challenges and provide for the high quality human caring in nursing.

Key Words: A super-aging society, Issues of healthcare, Issues of long-term care, Medical and welfare systems, Community-based integrated care systems

Chapter I

Japan's Super-aging Society and Situational Concerns

in Providing a High Quality Human Care System

By Mitsuko Omori

Chapter I

1. Introduction

With the low birth rate and the extended life span of Japanese people, it is estimated that those over the age of 65 accounted for 26% of the population in 2014. By 2025, this is anticipated to increase to about 30%, and to about 40% in 2060. The increase in the aging population has a strong impact on the nation's social security system, including the medical insurance and nursing care insurance systems. The deterioration of social security financing due to smaller contributions from a reduced working-age population affects the provision of benefits in the medical care system. Nevertheless, the aging population requires the increase in demand for healthcare and long-term care services. Japan's problems regarding the care of the super-aged citizens, the increase in social security costs, and the reduction of the working-age population have increased the worker care burden, and continue to strain the healthcare insurance systems [1-4].

The super-aged population lives long and healthy lives partly due to excellent medical care, technological advances in medicine, and improved nutritional status. It is clearly important that the quality of life of the older adults is regarded as most important to Japanese society, for they enrich the social classes due to their longer lives. As such, with an older adult population, the normal perspective on life-span development is often focused on having a full life until death. Young people need to appreciate the value of living longer while enjoying the fruits of their labors. However, this does not always seem logical. While the older adults live long and healthy lives, Japanese society aims to have their people and their social class surroundings support the governance of organizations through government entities and private foundations, so they could live a life full of hope, happiness, and care.

2. Current status and future of Japan's aging population

In 2007, the Japanese society became super-aged. The older adult population was 7% in 1970, but in 1994, the population of older adults doubled, and in 2007, the

3

Part 1

older adult population made up 21%. Japan became a "super-aged" society, and is now facing a population of super-aged persons more than any other country in the world.

The total population of Japan was 127.08 million people as of October 1, 2014. The number of people aged 65 and over is the highest ever, at 33 million. The percentage of the older adult population is now 26.0%. Of people aged 65 and over, the number of males was 14.23 million and women 18.77 million. The population of those aged 65-74 years old is 17.08 million; those 75 years old and over is 15.92 million people comprising 13.4% and 12.5% of the total population, respectively [5].

A long-term population decline will continue so that Japan will have less than 120 million people by 2026, 100 million by 2048, until the total population of Japan will be estimated to reach 86.74 million by 2060. In the future, as the total population decreases, the percentage of the elderly will continue to increase [5].

In 2015, when the baby boomers (born between from 1947 to 1949) begin reaching 65 years old, the number of elderly persons will grow to 33.95 million and will further increase. As the elderly population reaches its peak of 38.78 million in 2042, the percentage of the elderly will have greatly increased. In 2060, the percentage of the elderly will reach 39.9% with 1 in 2.5 people being 65 years and over. Also, the percentage of people aged 75 and over will be 26.9%, with 1 in 4 being 75 years and over [5].

If the burden of people who are paying into the public nursing care insurance system is increasing in this situation, beneficiaries of life, medical care and welfare systems of the elderly in the future will be difficult to obtain. With a declining birthrate and marriage rate, it is necessary to create a civil infrastructure for child care support and a comfortable working environment for mothers with children. For the increased population of the elderly aged 75 years or over, it is important to cooperate closely with medical and welfare systems, in which measures of preventive healthcare becomes mandatory in order to extend their healthy life expectancy.

It's vital to create an enabling environment for the elderly to continue to work as well as young people; also, it is necessary to change people's mindset about working.

Currently, as of 2013, the life expectancy at birth is 80.21 years for male and 86.61 years for female. By 2060, it will be 84.19 years for male and 90.93 years for female (exceeding 90 years old for female) [3].

There are two factors that influence the increase in a super-aging society: (1) an increase of the 65-year-old population due to a decrease in mortality, and (2) a reduction of the young population due to declining birthrates. In 2015, there were 2.3 persons of working age (aged 15-64) per elderly person. In 2060, there will be 1.3 persons of working age (aged 15-64) per elderly person. The arrival of a society where 1.3 persons of working age support an elderly person [5] is just around the corner.

In 2015, the number of births was 1,005,677, which continues to decrease, until it is estimated to decrease by about 24 million people in 2060, and less than or equal to half of that number in terms of the years of the younger population that will become the future production-based or working-age population [6]. Japan's declining birthrate and aging population increased the number of elderly persons. However, there is a shortage of people to support these elderly persons, increasing the possibility of a serious healthcare and social problem (Fig. 1-1).

Part 1

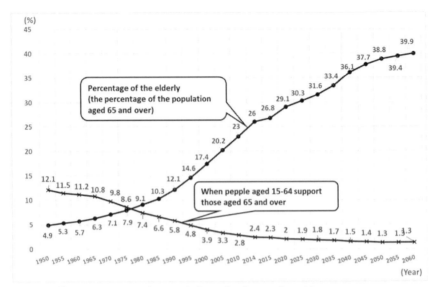

Fig. 1-1: Future prospects in population of aging and working age

(This figure was prepared from the information of the source:

http://www8.cao.go.jp/kourei/english/annualreport/2014/pdf/c1-1.pdf)

3. Robotic solution in nursing care work

The use of robotic technology in the healthcare field is strongly desired to relieve the burden of nursing-care workers. To overcome expected obstacles, the Ministry of the Economy, Trade and Industry of Japan has identified the following key goals: Identify key development areas based on actual needs [needs-oriented]; improve ease of use and lower costs through stage-gate trials [low cost]; solicit public and institutional support in order to implement the equipment at actual sites [large quantity]. To achieve these goals, the Ministry began the "Robotic Care Equipment Development and Introduction Project" beginning in 2013 until 2018. The Ministry of the Economy, Trade, and Industry and the Ministry of Health, Labour, and Welfare has formulated and released funding schemes. It is envisioned that supporting the development and introduction of robotic care equipment in the essential areas and creating a new market for robotic care equipment will partially lift the burden of care workers and empower those who require care. The key development areas and a list of scheduled and adopted robotic care equipment [7-10] are shown (Fig. 1-2).

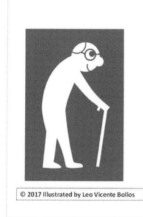

For elderly persons:
- **Monitoring systems for nursing care homes or private homes**
- **Outdoor or indoor mobility aids**
- **Toileting and bathing aids**

For care givers:
- **Wearable or non-wearable transfer aids**

Fig. 1-2: Key development areas of robotic care equipment

There is a developmental urgency to conduct empirical studies regarding the introduction of nursing care robots to Japanese society. Although this was initially difficult to advance, it is expected that with empirical studies, the introduction of robots in healthcare will become a reality. It is expected that robotic technology will lead to the aggressive use of robots, such as enhancing a sense of independent life for the elderly, awareness of health and prevention of low back pain for caregivers, and enriching the quality of human life.

Part 1

4. The environment surrounding the situation of medical treatment and care of the elderly

Based on the health conditions of the elderly aged 65 and over, the number of those experiencing adverse effects in their daily life was about 30%, in 2013. The ratio is higher for those in their late seventies and older. However, there are gender differences in that the number of women suffering these adverse effects is higher than men. The impact of age on the "activities of daily living", "work, housework and academic", "going out", "exercise" was seen in about 10% of the elderly [5].

The proportion of elderly people who receive medical treatment is higher than those of other ages. The number of hospitalized elderly with "cerebrovascular accident", "malignant neoplasm (cancer)" and "heart disease" is greater than those of younger age. The data on deaths among the elderly suggests that the highest rate of death (ratio of the number of deaths per elderly population of 100,000) among the elderly in 2013 was those caused by malignant cancers, numbering at 947.0, followed by heart diseases at 561.0 and pneumonia at 375.0 [5].

In particular, the elderly with dementia are highly likely to require increased nursing care. In 2012, the number of patients with dementia and the prevalence of those who were more than 65 years old with dementia was 4.62 million people, i.e. one person in seven persons (prevalence 15.0%). In 2025, the number of patients with dementia will increase to about 7 million people in a year, and roughly one in five people over 65 years of age are estimated to have dementia [6]. The number of people aged 65 and over who are certified as requiring long-term care is 5.457 million as of the end of fiscal year 2012, an increase of 2.580 million from the end of fiscal year 2001 (Fig. 1-3). The percentage of people who received the certification requiring long-term care in those 65-74 years of age (3.0%) and over 75 years of age (23.0%), and those more than 75-years-old has greatly increased [5].

8

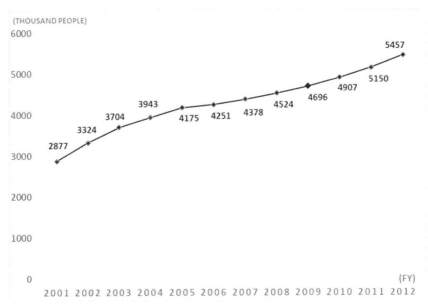

Fig. 1-3: Number of primary insured persons (aged 65 and over) requiring long-term care or support by care level

(This figure was prepared from the information of the source:

http://www8.cao.go.jp/kourei/english/annualreport/2014/pdf/c1-2-2.pdf)

A focus on the relationship of caregivers of elderly persons will show that more than 60% of them are living together with the persons receiving care. The main breakdown of caregivers is as follows: spouse (26.2%), children (21.8%), children's spouse (11.2%), and in a breakdown by gender: male (31.3%) and female (68.7%). As for the age of main caregivers living with the recipient, 69.0% of male and 68.5% of female caregivers were 60 years old and over, showing that family members, especially women, are the main caregivers with considerable cases falling into the category of those who "care for the elderly and are elderly themselves" [5]. In this way, the family supporting the elderly will have many elderly people to support, making it more difficult. Thus, abuse can occur because of the mental and physical burden of care, and it should be noted that there is a great possibility that murders or

Part 1

attempted suicides may become common [11-13]. Allowing comfortable "care for the elderly by the elderly" is necessary, and so the introduction of nursing care robots to assist in home care, thus reducing the caregivers' mental and physical burden, must be considered.

There were 101,100 women caregivers in 2011. Due to job changes, the number of women was reduced to 81,200, accounting for 80.3% of the total number. Separating by gender, age, turnover, and job change of men and women in their 50s and 60s shows that they accounted for about 70% of the caregiver population [6]. This means that, for long-term care among those who are burdened – even if not economically faced with physical and psychological aspects – the working population continues to decrease. In addition, about half of people who quit their jobs for the sake of long-term care claimed, "I wanted to continue to work". Reasons for the turnover included: "nursing care required a difficult workplace", "deterioration of their physical and mental health", "desire to concentrate on helping with their long-term care", and "if anyone cannot help, care burden increased" [6].

The main long-term caregivers who are living together and have the time required for care during the whole day come to about 40%. At the nursing care level, 4 or more, or about half of the primary caregivers have been providing care almost daily. Those whose care location is in the "home" account for about 40% of men and women, 30% of which being caregivers. Households with elderly people comprised 40% of the total population, with individuals living alone or households with a married couple holding a majority. The number of elderly people living alone is on the rise [5]. When the future elderly increase in number, the situation of need will become more and more long-term, and will eventually make it difficult for the family members to continue to work because of their loved ones' need for long-term care. "Care for the elderly by the elderly" and for the elderly without a caregiver are considered most likely to increase. The hope of the elderly who want to spend their lives at home would end up difficult.

Rapid aging is considered a major influential factor impacting the country's social security system, including medical insurance and nursing care insurance. The

Chapter I

elderly have more medical needs because of susceptibility to more than one chronic disease, dementia or disability, and because of growing needs such as physical care and close observation to persons who wander. As more people become elderly, the percentage of patients receiving care certification will increase. There is a great possibility that the shortage of people involved in healthcare will be much greater in the far future.

5. Elderly health and welfare systems

5.1. Medical insurance

Japan has a national health-insurance system that covers all of its citizens, and excellent public healthcare services, helping the nation achieve the world's highest average life expectancy and a low infant mortality rate. Because of the rapidly declining birthrate and simultaneously increasing aging population, the need for a Community-Based Integrated Care Systems (CBICS) becomes all the more critical so that it can foster needed changes in the medical and welfare fields. The medical care comprehensive system ensured by the Promotion Law was established in 2014, positioning the subjects of regional medical concepts, differentiation and the coordination of the feature of hospital beds, enhancements such as home care, and the reform of the healthcare delivery system [14]. Also in the medical insurance system, efforts to meet the challenges of the financial front were realized. For example, financial systems of prefectures and municipalities and their roles in national health insurances, review of medical benefit costs for the elderly, and promotion of prevention and health promotion have been studied.

5.2. Long-term care insurance system

In 2000, the long-term care insurance system was created as a mechanism to support care for the elderly [1]. Core city and municipal governments that have been designated and supervised for the need of long-term care services in prefectures and ordinance-designated cities were instituted. For the services making long-term care

11

Part 1

benefits available in the house and facilities, services for the prevention benefits in such settings, services for outpatient and short-term residents in the prefectures and ordinance-designated cities, core cities are performing the designation and supervision. The community-based care services, preventive care services, and preventive care assistance have designated municipalities for supervision [15].

The certified number of people requiring long-term care as of 2012 was 5.457 million people. This has increased by about 1.90-fold in the last 12 years [5]. The pace of increase in long-term care certification in recent years has been expanding. A long-term care insurance system has been established as necessary for the care of the elderly. Considering the progress of aging among Japan's "baby boomers" means that by 2025, when they become 75 years of age or more, the ratio will become one to 5.5 persons. Similarly, the number of elderly people with dementia is projected to increase [5]. If the people and their families in need of care wish to receive care at home, it is important to build optimal "CBICS" with features based on the elderly's healthcare needs.

5.3. Establishment of community-based integrated care systems

"Elderly people want to live a meaningful life with dignity until the end of their lives, but in their own homes, as much as possible".

This desire is common to many elderly people. But even if the situation of the elderly becomes severe up to the point of requiring nursing home care, it remains critical that such a desire can be fulfilled. It is their hope.

However, there are big regional differences regarding situations consequent to aging. The "CBICS" can provide the elderly – depending on the circumstances of the community and according to their abilities – the means to remain independent as long as possible. Therefore, the goal of the CBICS is to ensure that the elderly are able to sustain independent daily living, to possess medical care, nursing care, preventive care, shelter and independent support of everyday life [14]. Because of such a state of community resources and the increasing aging population, it is important to construct the CBICS according to their respective and allowable regional circumstances.

Chapter I

Effective CBICS construction will include the promotion of home care and nursing care cooperation, dementia measures, community care conference, enhancement and strengthening of life support services, prevention benefits, and support of regional business and nursing home residents. In principle, the CBICS is focused on continuing the nursing care insurance system, such as ensuring fairness and welfare and relieving nursing care personnel of care burden [1]. With further aging and population decline, in the future the foundations of medical and nursing care services will become an urgent issue to secure the human resources for the CBICS. By 2030, 16-17% of the total number of workers will be expected to work in the medical and welfare field, while it is estimated that 20-25% of the population will be qualified to receive such care.

The population of working-age people will be reduced because gathering the human resources needed for healthcare and long-term care, and ensuring human resources will be difficult. Along with the ongoing training of medical and nursing care personnel, turnover and latent prevention and re-employment of support are essential to ensure effective human resources [4]. Japan is also promoting acceptance of human resources from abroad. Based on the Economic Partnership Agreement (EPA), Japan has started to accept Indonesian, Filipino, and Vietnamese candidates in the field of nursing and nursing care on an annual basis since 2008. Every year, more than a dozen to hundred candidates from each country are learning and working in Japan. However, their passing rate for the national examination is quite low, which is a huge problem [16-19].

In addition to strengthening the foundations of medical and nursing care, securing human resources is another issue: the direction of future studies of the Ministry of Health, Labor and Welfare, while firmly responsive to the needs of the growing medical and welfare fields will try to build a system for creating a virtuous cycle of the economy at the same time. In order to do it, not only the training of new personnel, but also innovation in the field level such as business efficiency (to actively take advantage of the creation of new work environments), robots and ICT (Information and Communication Technology) must work [10, 20].

13

Part 1

The nursing home is in a dire situation in that the new residents have become qualified to a level of care that is 3 levels higher or more, in the revision of the long-term care insurance system. In level 3 persons are not able to care for themselves, particularly on grooming and maintaining personal belongings, including maintaining a clean living room. These persons cannot perform complicated actions such as rising from a sitting position and or using their legs to stand. They may have difficulty moving around independently, or standing on both feet. These persons cannot move their bowels and use the toilet by themselves, and oftentimes they have some behavioral problems and a steady decline in their total understanding.

In the nursing homes, the average level of care needed was 4 or 5, and average age was in the late 80s. For levels 4 and 5 the situation and condition of these persons are more severe than those persons in level 3: they can hardly do anything for themselves independently.

Currently, with insufficient manpower, nursing home care has become unsatisfactory because of the understaffing problem and staff who have not received adequate education. Some elderly welfare facilities are expected to introduce healthcare robots to counteract these problems and provide satisfactory nursing home care for their residents. To provide evidence for this type of solution, a study was conducted about the possibility of having robots in nursing homes.

To ensure the quality of life of the elderly in a small facility, the role of the robot was ensuring safety for all residents. The robot, instead of the staff, will watch over the elderly people with dementia to avoid the risk of wandering and falling. For example, when an elderly person with dementia wants to move, the robot can say "Just a moment, please. Please wait there. I have called the nurse who will be with you shortly", to help curb the risk of the elderly person falling when he or she stands up from the chair to go to the toilet. The robot can also sound the alarm to warn of impending problems, e.g. falls among the elderly population. In addition, when the elderly person with dementia becomes restless and wanders through the corridors, snuggles near, and with other patients, the robot can keep a close eye on them. At the same time, the robot can talk gently saying, "Now, it is night. Let's go back to your

14

Chapter I

room and have a rest". With a gentle voice, the robot can claim the attention of the elderly person, and the robot can inform the nursing staff that the elderly person is in danger.

The elderly can feel the special need to have a conversation partner, even if only a robot is available. The robot will know the elderly person's personality and hobbies, interests, and can converse to fit the content of the conversation, not only face-to-face, since the robot is able to produce a funny atmosphere if it is in a conversation with several people in the group. If the future robot is learning in an outstanding way, the robot can be a nice co-responder. Through the movement of the robot, nursing staff will be able to learn excellent ways of conversation together with robot activities and robot-to-human interactions.

In the hospital, there are also situations where a patient's dementia worsens, and a lot of manpower may be demanded. In the same way as humans watch over elderly people with dementia, provide risk aversion care treatments, and provide a conversation partner when required, an advanced practice could also be conceived to provide the necessary information to determine the staff to be involved in robot care. Robots will provide for the accumulated and complex needs of the patient, and check for careless mistakes – which can be expected – for example, to prevent the patient from falling into a rut.

6. Conclusion

Japanese society has become a super-aged society, one where the number of aging people is increasing rapidly. Japan's problems about the super-aged society are the expected increase in social security costs, the reduction of production population, and an increase in the care burden. Thus, with the aging of Japanese persons, there is a greater possibility of an increasing lack of people involved in the medical and nursing care fields to support a great deal of needs in the same areas. Therefore, in the areas of elderly health and its welfare system, medical insurance reform for long-term care insurance has promoted the construction of the CBICS.

15

Part 1

In order to promote the viability of the nursing care insurance system, construction of the CBICS ought to remain to ensure fairness and welfare among nursing care personnel, and to decrease the human care burden [21-24]. In the midst of a declining population, the development of alternative resources and the adjustment of the work environment also requires innovation in the field level, and the healthcare robot seems to be the partner in this endeavor.

References

[1]   Tsutsui T: Implementation process and challenges for the community-based integrated care system in Japan. Int J Integr Care, Vol. 14, No. 1, published online, 2014. DOI: 10.5334/ijic.988

[2]   Imai H: What problems will we confront in 2025? An analysis of public health and welfare issues. J. Natl. Inst. Public Health, Vol. 65, No. 1, pp. 2-8. 2016.

[3]   Arai H, Ouchi Y, et al.: Japan as the front-runner of super-aged societies, Perspectives from medicine and medical care in Japan. Geriatr Gerontol Int, Vol. 15, pp. 673-687, 2015. DOI: 10.1111/ggi.12450/pdf

[4]   Ministry of Health, Labour and Welfare Japan: Annual Health, Labour and Welfare Report 2015. http://www.mhlw.go.jp/english/wp/wp-hw9/index.html
(Accessed 12 November 2016)

[5]   Cabinet Office Japan: Annual Report on the Aging Society [Summary] FY 2015, The State of Aging and Implementation of the Measures for an Aging Society in FY, 2014. http://www8.cao.go.jp/kourei/english/annualreport/2015/2015pdf_e.html
(Accessed 20 September 2016)

[6]   Cabinet Office Japan: Annual Report on the Aging Society [Summary] FY 2016, The State of Aging and Implementation of the Measures for an Aging Society in FY 2015.
http://www8.cao.go.jp/kourei/whitepaper/w-2015/html/zenbun/s1_2_3.html
(Accessed 20 September 2016)

[7]   Robotic Care Devices Portal: Robotic Devices for Nursing Care Project.
http://robotcare.jp/?lang=en (Accessed 10 November 2016)

16

Chapter I

[8] Ministry of Economy, Trade and Industry: Joint Press Release with the Ministry of Health, Labour and Welfare, Revision of the Four Priority Areas to Which Robot Technology is to be Introduced in Nursing Care of the Elderly –Three priority items have been newly designated, including bathing–.
http://www.meti.go.jp/english/press/2014/0203_02.html
(Accessed 10 November 2016)

[9] Nursing Care and Robots: Ministry of Economy, Trade and Industry, Respond to actual needs with technology!
http://www.meti.go.jp/english/publications/pdf/journal2013_04.pdf
(Accessed 10 November 2016)

[10] Niimi Y: Global Dementia Legacy Event Japan New Care and prevention models.
http://www.ncgg.go.jp/topics/dementia/documents/Topic3-6YoshikiNiimi.pdf

[11] Salari S: Patterns of intimate partner homicide suicide in later life: Strategies for prevention. Clinical Interventions in Aging, Vol. 2, No.3, pp. 441-452, 2007.

[12] Bourget D, Gagné P, Whitehurst L: Domestic Homicide and Homicide-Suicide: The Older Offender. Journal of the American Academy of Psychiatry and the Law Online, Vol. 38, No. 3, pp. 305-311, 2010.

[13] Kishimoto Y, Terada S, et al.: Abuse of people with cognitive impairment by family caregivers in Japan (a cross-sectional study). Psychiatry Res. Vol. 209, No. 3, pp. 699-704, 2013.

[14] Ministry of Health, Labour and Welfare Japan: Long-Term Care Insurance System of Japan, Long-Term Care, Health and Welfare Services for the Elderly.
http://www.mhlw.go.jp/english/policy/care-welfare/care-welfare-elderly/dl/ltcisj_e.pdf (Accessed 12 November 2016)

[15] Ministry of Health, Labour and Welfare Japan: Health and Welfare Services for the Elderly, Long-Term Care, Health and Welfare Services for the Elderly.
http://www.mhlw.go.jp/english/wp/wp-hw9/dl/10e.pdf
(Accessed 12 November 2016)

[16] NPO/NGO CJWP ~ Connecting Japan With Philippines ~.
https://cjwp.amebaownd.com/ (Accessed 21 November 2016)

17

Part 1

[17] The Japan Foundation: Japanese-Language Pre-training Program for Indonesian and Filipino Candidates for Nurses and Care Workers under Economic Partnership Agreements (EPA). https://www.jpf.go.jp/e/project/japanese/education/training/epa/ (Accessed 21 November 2016)

[18] JAPAN TODAY: Indonesian, Filipino nurses to be allowed to stay extra year to pass exam. https://www.japantoday.com/category/national/view/indonesian-filipino-nurses-to-be-allowed-to-stay-extra-year-to-pass-exam (Accessed 21 November 2016)

[19] Ohno S: Southeast Asian Nurses and Caregiving Workers Transcending the National Boundaries: An Overview of Indonesian and Filipino Workers in Japan and Abroad. Southeast Asian Nurses, Vol. 49, No. 4, 2012.

[20] Miura K: Global Dementia Legacy Event Japan New Care and prevention models. http://www.mhlw.go.jp/english/policy/care-welfare/care-welfare-elderly/dl/141117-3.pdf (Accessed 14 November 2016)

[21] Maki Y, Yamaguchi H: Early detection of dementia in the community under a community-based integrated care system. Geriatr Gerontol Int, Vol. 14 (Suppl 2), pp. 2-10, 2014.

[22] Awata S: Toward the establishment of a community-based integrated care system supporting the lives of elderly patients with dementia. Japanese Journal of Geriatrics. Vol. 50, No. 2, pp. 200-204, 2013. (in Japanese)

[23] Japanese Nursing Association: Nursing in Japan 2016. https://www.nurse.or.jp/jna/english/pdf/nursing-in-japan2016.pdf (Accessed 14 November 2016)

[24] Naruki H: Examining the importance of and identifying methods to promote "integration" for structuring community-based integrated care systems. J. Natl. Inst. Public Health, Vol. 65, No. 1, pp. 47-55, 2016.

Abstract

This chapter introduces the key development areas of personal care robots, their required features, and meeting the International Organization for Standardization (ISO) 13482 as the international standard. As the top country for longevity, Japan faces challenges to enrich people's lives. One of the challenges is to put robotic technology to practical use in nursing. Based on this need, there are some research and development projects and international standards needed to support these projects focused on safety elements.

Key Words: Robotics features, Support for physical activities, Safety requirements, Personal care robots

Chapter II

Necessary Robotic Features to Support the Physical Activities and Rehabilitation of the Elderly

By Kazunori Yamazaki, Kenichi Sugawara, Soichiro Koyama, Shigeo Tanabe

Part 1

1. Introduction

Japan is facing severe socioeconomic pressures due to its aging and shrinking population. When the public nursing care insurance system for the elderly was introduced in Japan, there were approximately 550,000 nursing care workers in fiscal year (FY) 2000 [1]; in FY 2013, the Ministry of Health, Labor, and Welfare, reported this number had tripled to 1.71 million [1]. Although 2.53 million workers will be needed in FY 2025, a shortfall of ~ 380,000 is expected [1]. The population of elderly people requiring nursing care increases while the chronic manpower shortage continues. Recruiting sufficient numbers of nursing care workers has also become difficult because this profession has a heavy workload that is further associated with physical problems, e.g. back pain. The high workload in nursing homes, together with low job dissatisfaction and occupational burnout, affect the caregivers' ability to provide adequate care [2]. In addition, 80% of physical therapists have reported pain in their musculoskeletal system, with 40% complaining of pain in their hands, wrists, and shoulders [3].

Personal care robots can help reduce the burden on workers and prevent them from leaving their profession. Japan is well-known for its development of personal care robots, but end users have not been impressed with such products. The major problem is that the "companies developing the robots did not sufficiently incorporate the opinions of relevant people – some of their products were too large or too expensive and consequently not used" [4]. In light of such a situation, the Ministries of Economy, Trade, and Industry and Health, Labor, and Welfare conducted a survey to identify the need for robot technology in nursing care. According to this survey, the ministries have revised the priority areas so as to deal with the requirements of caregivers for home nursing, patients with dementia, and other cases [5]. In FY 2014, the ministries started to support the development of such robots in the newly designated priority areas [5].

Chapter II

2. Key development areas of personal care robots

The Ministries of Economy, Trade, and Industry and Health, Labor, and Welfare designated eight priority areas related to the development and commercialization of robots to support the physical activities of elderly persons [5]. Personal care robots can reduce the physical burden of caregivers and enhance the abilities of recipients. These robots split up into two groups. One group is designed to reduce the physical burden of caregivers: they come as wearable or non-wearable transfer aids, toileting aids, bathing aids, and monitoring systems for nursing care homes or private homes. The other is designed to enhance the abilities of elderly recipients or users: outdoor or indoor mobility aids.

2.1. Wearable transfer aids

These are devices that are worn by a caregiver and use robotic technologies to provide powered assistance to the wearer [6]. Its main purpose is to alleviate physical burden on the caregivers during care activities. Transfer movement is a particularly frequent activity, and caregivers have to bear a heavy physical burden. Since the physical burden on the caregiver's lumbar region causes back pain, it is important that reducing the burden becomes the priority development goals. Also, in order to enhance the practicality of the device, it is necessary to have a structure that allows equipment to be self-detachable and user friendly. It must also be a structure that can be used between a bed, a wheelchair, and a toilet bowl for the efficient transfer assistance for the elderly person.

An example of this type is the robot suit HAL (CYBERDYNE, Inc.) [7]. This device minimizes the risk of back injuries by reducing the load on the back, using the control technology which responds to weak biopotential signals from the user's skin surface. The device understands their intentions, and provides the necessary assistance to make the intended motion. This device improves the work environment at hospitals, nursing homes, etc. by helping people to perform a task with reduced effort.

21

Part 1

A second example is the muscle suit for nursing care (Kikuchi Seisakusho Co., Ltd.) [8]. The light-weight, high-power suit provides artificial muscles powered by compressed air, and assists caregivers in performing tasks that place a heavy load on their back, such as moving a person from a bed to a bath. The user is free to move around, carrying just a tank of compressed air on their back with no additional cables. The suit turns on by reacting to the way the user breathes, which leaves both hands free for the task.

2.2. Non-wearable transfer aids

Non-wearable transfer aids use robotic technologies and provide powered assistance to a caregiver during lifting motions [9]. Regarding the specifications of the equipment, there are types that completely compensate for the burden on caregivers during transfer assistance, and types that partially compensate. The hanging-type transfer lifts include non-wearable type transfer aid equipment. In order to enhance the practical use of this equipment, it is important that it can be operated by one person even while assisting to transfer a person in need of care: it can be used by transferring persons between a bed with high frequency of assistance, and a wheelchair; and it requires such a device does not require additional work for its installation, such as building a foundation for the device, in order to have a structure that can be used by the single device/equipment.

As an example, transfer support robot Hug T1 has been proposed (Fuji Machine Mfg. Co., Ltd.) [10]. Hug was designed to support people with mobility issues, e.g. those having difficulty moving from a bed to a wheelchair, or a wheelchair to a toilet seat. Hug provides assistance to a person when moving to a sitting position or when a person needs to stand for a period of time, e.g. getting dressed. Hug supports individuals who can stand on their own, but have limited mobility when standing.

A second example is the rise-assisting bed (Panasonic Corporation) [11]. This robotic bed can be operated by one person and helps move a patient easily, safely, and smoothly. It has the features of an electronic full-reclining wheelchair and an

Chapter II

electronic care bed. The bed moves the patient without lifting them up, thereby ensuring patient safety and removing the fear of falling. Its ease of operation enables a caregiver to focus on the patient during transfer, which also ensures patient safety. Only one user is required to connect or separate the bed and a wheelchair. By applying robotic technology, different structures have been fused into a compact electronic reclining wheelchair and an electronic care bed, eliminating the need to carry a patient and creating a new type of wheelchair-bed that can move patients.

As one last example, the transfer aid device has been proposed (YASKAWA Electric Corporation) [12]. This bed-to-chair transfer aid was designed to reduce the physical burden of caregivers and help low-mobility individuals who spend long periods in bed to enjoy activities and socializing. Its easy operation and simple transfer mechanism allows a single helper to move a care-receiver from a bed to a wheelchair. Caregivers do not feel any physical stress when transferring the care receiver, thanks to the power-assisted robotic arms that do much of the lifting. The system uses a sling seat that provides stable support throughout a lifting action regardless of the care-receiver's bodily features. The robot provides posture support to the care receiver to help them prepare for subsequent actions after their transfer. It also controls pelvic inclination, which helps to seat the care receiver in the correct position. The robot assists with a gentle, smooth transfer so that the care receiver can just sit and relax during every ride. The structure is sturdy and stable so that it does not wobble even when the care receiver moves during transfer, thus avoiding physical or mental stress. An intuitive operation system makes the caregiver feel as if they actually were holding and helping move the person up or down.

2.3. Outdoor mobility aids

This category includes mobility support equipment and walking support devices that provide mobility and luggage assistance to the elderly outside their home [13]. However, since these mobility aids only refer to wheeled equipment that supports walking outdoors, they excludes rideable devices. Its structure, in order to enable independent use outdoors, may require more than four wheels, with a wheel

23

diameter that can be firmly moved even in rough terrain. Also, as a mechanism to assist the propulsion force on the uphill slope and the braking force on the descending slope, it is necessary to install a manual brake mechanism for safety. In order to improve its practical utility, it must also have a load-carrying function such as a loading platform that can be used to put this device into a car or the trunk of a normal-sized car using a standard folding mechanism. Similarly, to make the device functional, it should come at a weight (about 30 kg) that a caregiver can lift, and it should have a waterproof function so that trouble does not occur even if it happens to be left outdoors in bad weather.

As an example, the walking assist cart has been proposed (RT. WORKS Co., Ltd.) [14]. The assist brake control of this walking aid takes into consideration the road environment and operating force of the user. The cart operates in accordance with the pace of the user, thereby greatly reducing the risk of falling. It learns its operational characteristics from the physical condition of the user; therefore, anyone can use this walking aid in a comfortable manner. By utilizing network connections, monitoring is possible using walking history management where the information gathered by the sensors can be applied to healthcare applications.

A second example is the otasuke walker (Azbil Co., Ltd.) [15]. This walking aid provides physical and mental assistance to elderly people by making it easier for them to walk outdoors. The power assist operation automatically detects a slope, so the user does not feel the weight of the walker. As the structure of this device is based on a walker that is already on the market, users are familiar with the use of its handle, brake, seat, folding mechanism, etc. If it detects a condition that seems dangerous, it can call the user's family, thereby reducing the fear of going out unattended.

A third example is the walk assistance system considering movement on uneven terrain (IMASEN ENGINEERING CORPORATION) [16]. This device has a special mechanism that helps users to walk on uneven terrain and pass over steps on floors and streets, which commercial rollators find difficult. It provides load-reduction for hand baggage using electronic movement assistance and a basket.

Chapter II

It has a fall-prevention function that continually considers the environment during walking.

2.4. Indoor mobility aids

Indoor mobility aids help elderly and other physically challenged people get up and down and move around their home. These devices use robotic technologies and are specifically designed to assist users in going to the bathroom and sitting and standing up from a toilet unaided [17]. Its aim is for walking indoors that supports self-sustaining activities for persons who have declining gait and postural maintenance ability. Rideable type structure devices are excluded. The main aim of this device is to support the persons during walking attempts in their houses. However, it should be able to help the user get up from a chair-sitting position or a bedside-sitting position. Also, because it is intended for indoor use, there is a need to be able to use it in a standard-sized toilet rather than one requiring a special operation. As such, a series of toilet actions must be considered seriously, including many movements that can cause the posture to be unstable, such as standing upright from the toilet seat, attaching and detaching clothes, wiping oneself clean, turning direction inside the toilet.

As an example, mobility aid device has been proposed (YASKAWA Electric Corporation) [18]. This device was developed to help elderly people who are losing independent mobility by providing the support they need to move around indoors (particularly to get to the toilet). This goal is to help users improve their quality of life by assisting them in walking by themselves as much as possible. This mobility aid device helps users to get up, walk, sit down on a toilet, and maintaining an optimal position while in the bathroom.

A second example is the walker with a powered standing-up assistance function (Mitsuba Corp.) [19]. This walker helps users to get up from a bedside, chair, couch, toilet, etc., and it can then be used as a regular walker. Its armrest is adjustable by a powered mechanism that raises or lowers it to the optimal height for the user. The small rear casters and low bottom frame allow the rear casters to slide

25

Part 1

under a bed, couch, or other household items; users can keep the walker in an easy-to-use position and raise themselves in a stable manner.

2.5. Toileting aids

Toilet aid devices should be movable and be placed anywhere in a user's room. The robotic technologies used in these devices should also be maximized for effective waste treatment [20]. Many care recipients have difficulty getting to the toilet, therefore toilet aid installations must consider the physical structures in the patient's room. However, when developing the toileting aids in order not to cause the odor annoyance of excrement, it is necessary to discharge the contaminants outside the room or confine these in a gas-tight container or bag.

As one example among many, the room-mounted mobile flush toilet has been proposed (TOTO Ltd.) [21]. This toilet is designed to be used in a user's private room. When the user is finished, the toilet flushes to clean the bowl and crushes and pressure-feeds the waste outside into the sewer system. This toilet uses flexible pipes on the floor for its plumbing system to ensure it can be moved as far as the pipes can reach. It also has lockable casters on the bottom that enable users to move it easily.

2.6. Bathing aids

Bathing aids are devices using robotic technologies to provide support for elderly people in the series of motions required for getting in and out of bathtubs [22]. This equipment includes not only specifications used by persons in need of nursing care but also specifications to be used with the assistance of other caregivers. As a required function, bathing aids help a series of bathing operations such as getting over the edge of the bathtub and standing upright in the bathtub. It is necessary to have a structure that can oblige the user to soak in the bathtub at least up to their chests. However, it must be realized that it is more difficult to care for patients at the deep end of the bathtub. Since narrow bathrooms are also used by family members of care recipients, a mechanism that allows the helper to easily store required paraphernalia for bathing in order not to disturb their bathing habits is

Chapter II

important. Moreover, it is important to note that special construction of bathing aids is unnecessary for this equipment.

2.7. Monitoring systems for nursing care homes

Equipment and platforms using sensors and external communication facilities that support the monitoring of patients at long-term care facilities are needed [23]. This support device is to ensure patient's safe living, unlike a device that supports patient's daily living activities itself. In welfare support equipment of this type of nursing care facility, it is possible to observe activity information of many patients at the same time and its information sharing can be easily done among caregivers within a facility. Especially, it is necessary to automatically and constantly monitor/detect the patient's act of leaving the bed as quickly as possible, and transmit this information to the caregivers daily.

It is not like a traditional "nurse call" device, like those that patients use – pressing a call button. This function is capable of alerting caregivers when the patient has left their bed or is trying to do so. In addition, various devices and software for expanding the watching/observation system have been commercialized; this device is required to be easy-to-use-to connect with external devices.

As an example, the non-contact tracking system for dementia patients used on beds using a vision sensor has been proposed (IDEAQUEST Co., Ltd.) [24]. The implementation of a completely non-contact and unrestrained sensing device ensures that the care receiver does not encounter any physical limitations when using this equipment. A neural network algorithm using three-dimensional reconstruction of the human body detects any dangerous position taken by the care receiver. Through an analysis of motion information obtained from the vision sensor, biological reactions can be detected (These detection rate of false alarms are low.). The reaction time for the warning alarm is within 30 s or less in case of an emergency. External reports of the equipment are carried out only by telephone or through a nurse call system.

Part 1

2.8. Monitoring systems for private homes

Monitoring systems for private homes are devices and platforms that use robotic technologies with sensors and external communication functions to monitor the elderly and other persons [25]. While this system may be designed for one person, such as those with dementia or those with higher brain dysfunctions, it must also be understood that this system must be able to monitor multiple rooms at the same time. Even in bathrooms and dark places, this system is necessary to constantly detect the behavior style, physical condition change, and falling episodes of the care recipient, so it is undesirable to have the specification on the premise that the person carries it or wears it. With enhanced functions and additional devices and software, the devices have the potential to provide a platform to monitor patients with dementia.

As an example, the monitoring system using radar technologies (fall detector for private homes) has been proposed (CQ-S NET) [26]. This radar light system consists of a radar, light emitting diodes (LEDs), and a radio communication unit. It is designed to capture reflected waves with its built-in radar, to analyze them to detect the movements of a care receiver – such as getting up, leaving the bed, and falling – and send an alarm to a caregiver if necessary. The system is a non-contact device that is installed on the ceiling and requires no changes in the care receiver's living environment while offering constant monitoring services. The monitoring camera is built into the LED equipment attached to the ceiling, which eases the care receiver's discomfort at being watched continuously through conventional cameras and contributes to privacy protection. The built-in radar in the LED equipment enables non-contact measurements of the distance between the radar and care receiver and non-contact monitoring of their movements, and detects abrupt changes in position and motions, such as a fall or crouch. This system can monitor the care receiver 24 h a day regardless of their whereabouts at home and send an emergency alarm to portable devices such as a tablet computer.

28

Chapter II

3. ISO 13842 for the safety requirements for personal care robots

Personal care robots are a new technology expected to improve the quality of our lives in the foreseeable future. However, unlike industrial robots, these new robots require special safety features because of their immediate contact with human users. Therefore, the International Organization for Standardization (ISO) has developed an associated standard (ISO 13482) in recognition of the particular hazards presented by newly emerging "robots and robotic devices" [27]. ISO 13482 was realized based on proposals submitted to the ISO from Japan.

ISO 13482 focuses on the "safety requirements for personal care robots" in non-medical applications. This international standard complements ISO 10218-1 [28], which only covers the safety requirements for robots in industrial environments. This international standard includes additional information in line with ISO 12100 [29] and adopts the approach proposed in ISO 13849 [30-32] and International Electrotechnical Commission (IEC) 62061 to formulate a safety standard for robots and robotic devices in personal care to specify the conditions for physical human-robot contact. In the standard, personal care robots are classified into three types:

(1) Mobile Servant Robot: a personal care robot that is capable of traveling to perform serving tasks during interactions with humans, such as handling objects or exchanging information.

(2) Physical Assistant Robot: a personal care robot that physically assists a user to perform tasks by supplementing or augmenting personal capabilities.

(3) Personal Carrier Robot: a personal care robot that transports humans to an intended destination.

These robots typically perform tasks to improve the quality of life of the intended users, irrespective of age or capability.

29

Part 1

ISO 13482 describes the hazards associated with the use of these robots, and provides requirements to eliminate or reduce these risks to an acceptable level, and the international standard covers human-robot physical contact applications. This international standard does not apply to:

- robots travelling >20 km/h;
- robot toys;
- water-borne robots and flying robots;
- industrial robots, which are covered in ISO 10218;
- robots as medical devices;
- military or public force application robots.

However, the safety principles established in ISO 13482 can be useful for the robots listed above.

4. Conclusion

Safety verification, facility environment, and medical and engineering advice from developers must be secured as humans are now starting to use personal care robots. This will create a favorable cycle of development, support, and know-how, leading to the development of pragmatic robotic nursing care equipment. Conversely, others assert that it is only a matter of time before robots replace a host of other professions. According to a 2013 University of Oxford study [33], 50% of American jobs could be automated within the next 2 decades. However, robots do not yet have the ability to perform complex tasks such as negotiation or persuasion, and they are not as proficient in generating new ideas as they are at solving problems. This means jobs requiring creativity, emotional intelligence, and social skills are unlikely to be filled by robots any time soon [34]. Therefore, it is likely that nurses and nursing care workers will remain human for the foreseeable future. Personal care robots can only reduce the physical burden of caregivers and enhance the abilities of recipients, but despite this limitation, they still can provide opportunities to improve lives. We

Chapter II

are looking forward to the new age of nursing care in Japan, because a healthy life expectancy begins here.

References

[1] Ministry of Internal Affairs and Communication, Statistics Bureau: Statistical Handbook of Japan, Chapter 15: Social Security, Health Care, and Public Hygiene. http://www.stat.go.jp/english/data/handbook/ (Accessed 22 November 2016)

[2] Bae YH, Lee JH, Yoo HJ: Associations between work-related musculoskeletal pain, quality of life and presenteeism in Physical Therapists. J Korean Soc Occup Environ Hyg, Vol. 22, pp. 61-72, 2012.

[3] Hwang HL, Hsieh PF, Wang HH: Taiwanese long-term care facility residents' experiences of caring: a qualitative study. Scand J Caring Sci, Vol. 27, No. 3, pp. 695-703, 2013. DOI: 10.1111/j.1471-6712.2012.01082.x

[4] Robotic Devices for Nursing Care Project: Robotic Care Devices Portal: Implementing Nursing Equipment in the Real World. http://robotcare.jp/?lang=en (Accessed 22 November 2016)

[5] Ministry of Economy, Trade and Industry: Revision of the Four Priority Areas to Which Robot Technology is to be Introduced in Nursing Care of the Elderly. http://www.meti.go.jp/english/press/2014/0203_02.html (Accessed 22 November 2016)

[6] Robotic Devices for Nursing Care Project: Robotic Care Devices Portal: Wearable transfer aids. http://robotcare.jp/?page_id=29&lang=en (Accessed 22 November 2016)

[7] CYBERDYNE inc.: HAL for Labor Support. https://www.cyberdyne.jp/english/products/Lumbar_LaborSupport.html (Accessed 22 November 2016)

[8] Kikuchi Seisakusho Co., Ltd.: Muscle Suit. http://www.kikuchiseisakusho.co.jp/mechatro2/RobotTechnology.html (Accessed 22 November 2016) (in Japanese)

31

Part 1

[9] Robotic Devices for Nursing Care Project: Robotic Care Devices Portal: Non-wearable transfer aids.

http://robotcare.jp/?page_id=38&lang=en (Accessed 22 November 2016)

[10] Fuji Machine Mfg. Co., Ltd.: Transfer Support Robot Hug.

http://nfa.fuji.co.jp/e/products/Hug/detail.php?id=2 (Accessed 22 November 2016)

[11] Panasonic Corporation: Rise Assisting Bed – Resyone.

http://www.panasonic.com/jp/company/ppe/resyone.html

(Accessed 22 November 2016) (in Japanese)

[12] YASKAWA Electric Corporation: YASKAWA Report 2015.

https://www.yaskawa.co.jp/en/wp-content/uploads/2015/01/ar2015_E.pdf

(Accessed 22 November 2016)

[13] Robotic Devices for Nursing Care Project: Robotic Care Devices Portal: Outdoor mobility aids.

http://robotcare.jp/?page_id=42&lang=en (Accessed 22 November 2016)

[14] RT.WORKS: Robot assist walker RT1. https://www.rtworks.co.jp/product/rt1.html

(Accessed 22 November 2016) (in Japanese)

[15] Robotic Devices for Nursing Care Project: Robotic Care Devices Portal: Otasuke Walker (Azbil Co., Ltd.). http://robotcare.jp/?page_id=863&lang=en

(Accessed 22 November 2016)

[16] Robotic Devices for Nursing Care Project: Robotic Care Devices Portal: Walk assistance system considering steps on the ground and uneven terrain (IMASEN ENGINEERING CORPORATION). http://robotcare.jp/?page_id=865&lang=en

(Accessed 22 November 2016)

[17] Robotic Devices for Nursing Care Project: Robotic Care Devices Portal: Indoor mobility aids. http://robotcare.jp/?page_id=1940&lang=en

(Accessed 22 November 2016)

[18] YASKAWA Electric Corporation: YASKAWA Report 2016.

https://www.yaskawa.co.jp/en/wp-content/uploads/2016/08/ar2016_E-35-36.pdf

(Accessed 22 November 2016)

[19] Robotic Devices for Nursing Care Project: Robotic Care Devices Portal: Walker with a powered standing-up assistance function (Mitsuba Corp.). http://robotcare.jp/?page_id=2310&lang=en (Accessed 22 November 2016)

[20] Robotic Devices for Nursing Care Project: Robotic Care Devices Portal: Toileting aids. http://robotcare.jp/?page_id=64&lang=en (Accessed 22 November 2016)

[21] TOTO Ltd: Room-mounted Mobile Flush Toilet. http://www.toto.co.jp/products/ud/bedsidetoilet/index.htm (Accessed 22 November 2016) (in Japanese)

[22] Robotic Devices for Nursing Care Project: Robotic Care Devices Portal: Bathing aids. http://robotcare.jp/?page_id=1947&lang=en (Accessed 22 November 2016)

[23] Robotic Devices for Nursing Care Project: Robotic Care Devices Portal: Monitoring systems for nursing care homes. http://robotcare.jp/?page_id=68&lang=en (Accessed 22 November 2016)

[24] IDEAQUEST Inc.: Non-contact and non-constraint bedside safety monitoring systems, Owlsight for social welfare. http://www.ideaquest4u.com/english/products/products01/ (Accessed 22 November 2016)

[25] Robotic Devices for Nursing Care Project: Robotic Care Devices Portal: Monitoring systems for private homes. http://robotcare.jp/?page_id=1945&lang=en (Accessed 22 November 2016)

[26] Robotic Devices for Nursing Care Project: Robotic Care Devices Portal: Monitoring system using radar technologies (CQ-S NET). http://robotcare.jp/?page_id=2336&lang=en (Accessed 22 November 2016)

[27] ISO 13482:2014, Robots and robotic devices – Safety requirements for personal care robots. https://www.iso.org/obp/ui/#iso:std:iso:13482:ed-1:v1:en

[28] ISO 10218-1:2011, Robots and robotic devices – Safety requirements for industrial robots – Part 1: Robots. https://www.iso.org/obp/ui/#iso:std:iso:10218:-1:ed-2:v1:en

Part 1

[29] ISO 12100:2010, Safety of machinery – General principles for design – Risk assessment and risk reduction.
https://www.iso.org/obp/ui/#iso:std:iso:12100:ed-1:v1:en

[30] ISO 13849-1, Safety of machinery – Safety-related parts of control systems – Part 1: General principles for design. https://www.iso.org/obp/ui/#iso:std:69883:en

[31] ISO 13849-2, Safety of machinery – Safety-related parts of control systems – Part 2: Validation. https://www.iso.org/obp/ui/#iso:std:53640:en

[32] IEC 62061:2012, Safety of machinery – Functional safety of safety-related electrical, electronic and programmable electronic control systems. https://webstore.iec.ch/publication/6426

[33] Frey CB, Osborne MA: The future of employment: How susceptible are jobs to computerization? 2013.
http://www.oxfordmartin.ox.ac.uk/downloads/academic/The_Future_of_Employment.pdf (Accessed 22 November 2016)

[34] Huston C: The Impact of Emerging Technology on Nursing Care: Warp Speed Ahead. Online J Issues Nurs, Vol. 18, No. 2, p. 1, 2013.
DOI: 10.3912/OJIN.Vol18No02Man01

34

Abstract

This chapter introduces three types of activity assist robots for healthcare and rehabilitation: exercise assist robots, independence assist robots, and care assist robots. Future population projections indicate that the population in Japan will shrink by 2050, while the number of elderly will increase. The working age population will also drop, affecting the number of care-givers needed. One way to deal with this issue is the application of robots in human healthcare.

Key Words: Healthcare, Robotics, Population reduction, Aging society

Chapter III

Demand for Human Healthcare and Robotic Rehabilitation Welfare Services among the Current Oldest and the Incoming Elderly in Japanese Society

By Abbas Orand, Kotaro Takeda, Shigeo Tanabe

Part 1

1. Introduction

The Statistics Bureau of the Ministry of Internal Affairs and Communications [1], have predicted that the total population and number of elderly individuals aged over 65 years in Japan will be approximately 37 and 97 million by 2050 [2], respectively. As the number of elderly increases, their total population increases reaching 38.8% by 2050. Furthermore, the aging of society will also result in an increase in the number of disabled persons [3], thereby increasing medical cost. In Japan, wherein the incidence of patients experiencing their first stroke will increase as the number of elderly grows, will result in a concomitant rise in physical disabilities [4]. Considering that age is a risk factor for stroke, the aging of the world population puts a large number of persons at risk. Stroke survivors need support for meeting their daily activities and maintaining their quality of life. They need regular and frequent therapy and assistance to cope with the aftereffects of stroke. The decrease in the working population – together with the need for devices that can carry out high-intensity and repetitive training – makes the field of robotics highly suitable for the successful care and rehabilitation of the elderly. Thus, many Japanese automotive and industrial robot makers have begun to develop various types of robots for healthcare and rehabilitation. Robots can deliver precise quantitative exercise, support, and care, which will be discussed in the following sections.

This chapter introduces three types of activity assist robots for healthcare and rehabilitation: exercise assist robots, independence assist robots, and care assist robots.

2. Exercise assist robots

Exercise is effective in improving motor and cognitive functions [5]. Exercise assist robots have been designed and developed for debilitated persons. TOYOTA Co. has developed Gait and Balance Exercise Assist Robots (GEAR and BEAR,

Chapter III

respectively). While the first robot assists the elderly with their exercises for walking, the second robot assists them with their exercises for balance. Honda Motor Co., Ltd. has also developed a walking exercise assist robot called Stride Management Assist System (SMAS), to be used by the elderly during walking. These three exercise assist robots are introduced in the following section.

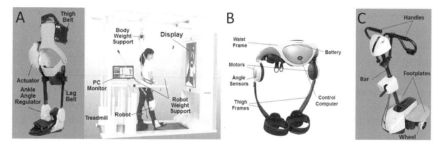

Fig. 3-1: A: **Gait Exercise Assist Robot (GEAR)**. This robot is equipped with an actuator at its knee that produces the required torque for flexion and extension. The robot is attached to two supporting wires at two points to compensate for its weight.

B: **Stride Management Assist System (SMAS)**. This system is available in three sizes: medium, large, and extra-large. It weighs 2.8 kg with its rechargeable ion battery. Two brushless DC motors with a maximum output torque of 4 Nm are used for its drive system. Angle and current sensors located in the motors allow the range of motion in degrees and torque to be monitored, respectively. The system can be operated for approximately 60 min with a single charge. Size-adjustable frames can be adopted so that people with various body sizes or types can use the system.

C: **Balance Exercise Assist Robot (BEAR)**. This robot has a two in-wheel-type design. Its dimensions are 480 × 700 × 1100 mm (W × L × H) and it weighs 21.3 kg.

37

Part 1

2.1. GEAR

In the GEAR system (Fig. 3-1: A) [6], a patient uses a treadmill to practice gait exercise. A large display is mounted in front of the patient so they can see the motion of their limbs or whole body during the exercise. A bodyweight support that is attached to the top of the structure keeps the patient from falling. The robot is secured to one of the patient's legs, and its weight is supported by two wires that are connected to the top of the system's steel structure. A computer and monitor are used to input and adjust the parameters of the system.

The concept behind the development of this system is to assist in the exercise of patients who suffer from hemi-lower limb paralysis resulting from stroke. The robot monitors the data generated during exercise – such as the angle of the knee – and is capable of providing sonic feedback to the patient receiving training. By assisting patients in extending their legs in an ordinary way and aiding them to support their own weight with the affected lower limb during extension of the unaffected knee, the robot helps the patients learn the normal pattern of walking.

Initially, a physician or a physical therapist sets the system's assistance parameters, according to the patient's requirements. As the training continues, the assistance from the robot is reduced. At this time, however, there are no published studies on the use or efficacy of the GEAR.

2.2. SMAS

SMAS was developed as an assistive wearable robotic device (Fig. 3-1: B) [7]. As an ambulation system it is worn around the hips to enhance the walking performance of the elderly and patients with a gait disorder by providing each hip joint with independent active flexion and extension capabilities.

This system assists independent hip flexion and extension by transmitting its generated torque to the thighs through thigh frames. A physician or a physical therapist can operate the system and a tablet computer can remotely modify its settings, even when the system is in use. A mutual rhythm scheme is used in the control architecture of SMAS to enhance the user's walking patterns [8]. The SMAS

Chapter III

controller synchronizes itself with the user's input using neural oscillators operating in conjunction with the user's central pattern generators, i.e. biological neural networks that generate rhythmic output patterns without sensory feedback [9]. The SMAS controller generates regulated walking patterns at specific instances during the gait cycle using the angle of sensors embedded in the actuators.

Three modes of "following", "symmetric", and "step" are available in SMAS [9]. In the "following" mode, SMAS assists the user's walking motions according to their walking pattern. Bilaterally symmetric motions, such as bending and extending both legs, are assisted by the robot in the "symmetric" mode. The "step" mode of SMAS assists the user to step repeatedly, enabling them to shift their weight smoothly.

The effects of SMAS have been investigated [9-11]. The application of SMAS to post-stroke individuals has led to reports of significant improvements of gait parameters [10]. In elderly individuals who used SMAS for a long time, one study showed that they could eventually walk with a wider stride, higher speed, and lower heart rate without assistance from the device [11].

2.3. BEAR

BEAR is a stand-up-and-ride robot (Fig. 3-1: C) [12]. In order to use the robot, the safety bar is first pushed down so that the end of the bar touches the floor and the robot is in a stable standing position. Then, the user stands on the two plates and grasps the handles attached to the bar at the center of the robot. After starting, the robot can move forward and backward as the user leans forward and backward, respectively. By shifting its weight to either left or right, the robot turns to the opposite side, as in skiing or skating. The robot uses the concept of an inverted pendulum system to stabilize itself [12]. The controller of the device constantly adjusts the device so that it does not fall. The controller is similar to a broom balanced in an inverted position [13]; to keep the broom upright, the user continually moves their hand in the same direction as the broom falls. By moving their hand to the other side of the broom's center of mass, the user generates torque that causes

39

Part 1

the broom to start falling in the opposite direction. The same motion of the hand in the opposite direction prevents the broom from falling and keeps it in an upright position.

Three specialized games, i.e., Tennis, Skiing, and Rodeo, have been developed to allow users to undergo balance training in an enjoyable manner. For the tennis game, the user is required to move a tennis player displayed on a screen in front of them forward or backward to return a tennis ball. For the skiing game, the user is required to turn a skier left or right to follow a ski course. And for the rodeo game, the user is required to remain in a standing position irrespective of disturbances. One can stop using the robot by pushing the safety bar downward until it makes contact with the floor. Then, the user can step off the machine.

One study [12] shows that the load placed on leg muscles can be adjusted by changing the degree of difficulty of the system's games. Another study [14] carried out two interventions of exercise against perturbation and exercise moving the center of gravity, which found that tandem gait speed, a functional reach test, functional base of support, and lower extremity muscle strength improved. The subjects of the study expressed their satisfaction with the balance exercises compared to conventional ones.

3. Independence assist robots

To support a better quality of life, different robots have been designed and developed. In this category of robots, the devices are not used to treat a condition, but to compensate for a user's dysfunctions by supporting their movement. Wearable Power-Assist Locomotor (WPAL), Walking Assist Robot (WAR), and Bodyweight Support System (BSS) are three independence assist robots that are introduced in this section.

Chapter III

3.1. WPAL

In order to assist paraplegic individuals with their gait, the WPAL system has been designed (Fig. 3-2) [15]. The concept of WPAL is to provide paraplegics with independent and comfortable walking. WPAL consists of two parts: robotics and orthotics. The user wears the orthosis for the majority of the time in a wheelchair and adds the robotic part when they wish to walk using a custom-made walker. The walker – weighing almost 12 kg – contains the batteries, control unit of the device, and buttons for selecting the different modes of the device. The walker is connected to the device through a cable. Under the regular gait condition, the power supply lasts for more than 1 h. In case of an emergency, a button on the hand grip of the walker allows the user to stop the device at any time.

WPAL has three gait modes and one sitting/standing mode. By triggering the sitting/standing mode, the user hears three beeps, after which WPAL assists the user either to sit or stand. After standing, the user can initiate standard gait mode by pressing the start button. Gait mode starts with three beeps and continues with sounds that correspond to the gait pattern. By using user-specific parameters, step length and step time are fixed, and the robot's controller initiates the motors of the three joints to fulfill the predetermined step length and step time. The two other gait modes of WPAL are "curve" and "slow". In "curve" mode, the user turns smoothly, which is achieved by keeping the step length of the foot on the outer side of the turning direction the same as during gait mode while shortening the step length of the foot on the inner side of the turning direction. On uneven surfaces, such as a road, "slow" mode is used.

Training with the device at five stages is required in order for the user to become acquainted with WPAL. This is necessary for the user to synchronize their rhythmic lateral weight shifts with those of the device. In the first stage, the user practices stepping in place. Gait exercise using a parallel bar is performed in the second stage. In the third and fourth stages, the user exercises with the device on a treadmill and then with a walker under a suspension system, respectively. In the fifth stage, the user practices gait with a walker but without suspension.

41

Part 1

One study [15] shows the superiority of WPAL to conventional orthoses in terms of physiological cost index, perceived exertion, and burden on the upper extremities. Another study [16] shows that the mean duration and distance of walking were higher than those of conventional orthoses.

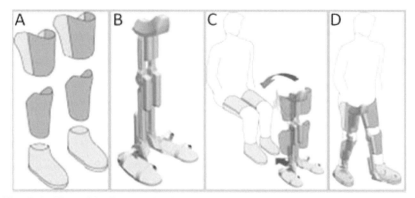

Fig. 3-2: **Wearable Power-Assist Locomotor (WPAL)** consists of two parts: orthotic (A) and robotic (B). The user wears the orthosis and adds the robotic part (C) for walking (D). Flexible cushions are used in the inner layer of the orthotic parts to avoid pressure sores. Rigid carbon plates stiffened by metal bars are used for the outer layers or parts. The orthotic parts weigh 4 kg. The robotic part weighs 9 kg and has 6 degrees of freedom (flexion-extension of bilateral hip, knee, and ankle joints). The maximum range of motion of the hip, knee, and ankle are 40° (flexion 25° and extension 15°), 120° (flexion 120° and extension 0°), and 50° (flexion35° and extension 15°), respectively.

Custom-made compact brushless DC motors (24 V, 78 W) are used at the three joints to enable each joint to flex or extend independently from the other two joints. The maximum peak torque of the motors is 30 Nm with a speed range between 0 and 1000 °/s. Joint angles are determined by resolvers built into the motors.

Chapter III

3.2. WAR

WAR is an assistive robot for persons with limited functionality in one leg caused by stroke or polio, for example. WAR was designed and developed by Toyota Co. (Fig. 3-3: A) [17]. The robot can be used after rehabilitation for typical daily activities such as walking on a level ground, climbing up and down stairs, standing up from or sitting on a chair, descending slopes, and climbing hills. WAR is attached to the affected leg and assists the user's walking. It has two sensors to detect the user's position and load on the thigh and on the sole of the foot, respectively. By using the data generated and assessing the user's stride, the actuator at the knee of the robot is regulated to provide the user with the best walking assistance. The assistance from WAR is produced in balance with the walking speed of the user, so that they can maintain the natural method of walking. WAR is powered by batteries that are packed in a bag worn by the user. Materials such as carbon fiber-reinforced polymer are used in WAR to keep its weight as low as possible, thus reducing its weight load.

3.3. BSS

BSS was designed and developed by Honda Motor Co., Ltd. (Fig. 3-3: B). The device was designed based on the concept of a "user-friendly walking assist device" assisting the user at their will [18]. The device provides an assistive force in parallel to a floor reaction force that extends from the bottom of the user's foot (center of pressure) to their center of gravity [18, 19]. When walking, the user exerts a force on the floor. The reaction force opposite to the floor force is the floor reaction force, which affects the leg muscles. By reducing the floor reaction force through the assistive force generated by the device, the effects on the muscles are reduced, resulting in a reduction of muscle activity and total body energy consumption [18]. The seat of the device, on which the groin of the user lies, receives the assistive force and transfers it to the user's center of gravity. The device is designed to keep the assistive force in the direction of the user's center of gravity, regardless of the position of the legs.

43

Part 1

A study on able-bodied subjects [18] measured the floor reaction force while the subjects walked slowly on a level ground with and without the device. Muscle activity and energy consumption were both reduced when the users adopted the device.

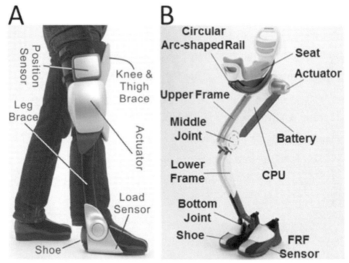

Fig. 3-3: A: **Walking Assist Robot (WAR)**. The WAR's dimensions are 280 × 290 × 620-770 mm (W × L × H) and it weighs 3.5 kg.

B: **Bodyweight Support System (BSS)**. BSS weighs 6.5 kg with its shoes and batteries. Two motors are used for its drive. A lithium ion battery is used for its power source and lasts for 2 h with a single charge.

4. Care assist robots

For relieving the burden on care-givers, engineers in cooperation with medical professionals have designed robots for the care of persons in need of assistance. Both of the robots introduced in this section were developed by TOYOTA Co. The

Chapter III

first robot is a Care Assist Robot (CAR) and the second one is a Human Support Robot (HSR).

4.1. CAR

CAR [17] is a combination of weight maintenance arms and an assisting chair (Fig. 3-4: A). The two arms are formed in such a way that they can fit easily between the arms and trunk of a person. By applying a very fine and detailed control algorithm and building compact control functionality, CAR embraces the individual in a comfortable and gentle manner. The robot is easy for a care-giver to use and it is gentle toward the care-receiver. The care-giver can, securely and gently, use the arms of the system to move the position of a person who has leaned against the main body of the robot. The care-giver can then easily move the robot to carry the individual to a desired location such as a toilet.

4.2. HSR

In order to assist with the independence of physically challenged persons, TOYOTA Co. has developed new technologies that are used in HSR (Fig. 3-4: B) [17]. TOYOTA has loaned its newly developed HSR to collaborating institutes for research purposes. These collaborating institutes will use the robot to promote the development of robotic technologies for the support of physically challenged persons and the elderly. By sharing HSR's software and hardware with the development community, TOYOTA intends to accelerate the improvement of this technology.

HSR has a flexible, cylindrical, small light-weight body that can store a moving arm. As a result, the robot is capable of picking up thin, hard-to-grip objects, such as paper or cards and also pens and TV remotes, and of removing objects from boxes and shelves by simply specifying what to fetch. The robot also has autonomous capabilities, which can be performed manually via the user interface. The manual control option allows care-givers and/or family members to communicate over the internet. Since its initial demonstration, TOYOTA has

45

Part 1

improved the functionality of HSR through assessment of the robot by care-giving professionals. The new HSR has improved in terms of functionality, safety, research development, and actual performance.

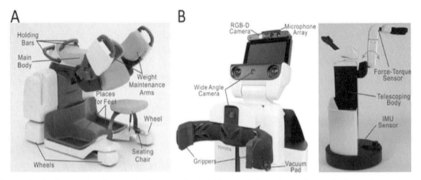

Fig. 3-4: A: **Care Assist Robot (CAR)**. CAR consists of a sitting chair and a robot, which has two weight maintenance arms. The individual is positioned on the seating chair and leans forward against the main body. They grasp the holding bars to secure their position. The care-giver controls both arms to hold the trunk of the individual gently from both sides. The care-giver can also move the main body up or down to keep the care-receiver in a secure position. The whole robot can be moved easily in any direction specified by the care-giver. The robot's dimensions are 700 × 995 × 900 mm (W × L × H) and it weighs 140 kg.

B: **Human Support Robot (HSR)**. HSR is capable of omnidirectional movements and its peak velocity is 0.8 km/h. Its telescopic body can reach a height of 135 cm and its minimum height is 100.5 cm. The diameter of HSR is 43 cm and it weighs 37 kg. The moving arm can rotate vertically; it is 60 cm long and its joints contain compliant controls.

Chapter III

5. Conclusion

The aging society and its extended life expectancy have increased the number of people in need of care and rehabilitation, while the number of working persons has decreased, making the integration of robotics into rehabilitation and care more feasible and desirable. The application of robotics as an adjunct to conventional rehabilitation has shown promising results. Robots are now more adaptable to the movements of patients as a result of technological advances and they can deliver repetitive, highly accurate training and exercises. However, the application of robots alone is not the solution for the care and rehabilitation of the elderly at the present time [20] because they are not cost-effective.

Overall, the common application of robots for the elderly is in its early stage. The advancement of technologies can help to build robots in more compact sizes and at affordable prices so that their use will not be limited to clinical applications, which will make robots more acceptable. The progress of technologies in engineering, computer science, and healthcare will make the field of robotics a promising solution for the problems of the elderly.

References

[1] Ministry of Internal Affairs and Communication, Statistics Bureau: Japan Statistical Yearbook, Chapter 2: Population and Households.
http://www.stat.go.jp/english/data/nenkan/1431-02.htm
(Accessed 28 October 2016)

[2] Ministry of Internal Affairs and Communication, Statistics Bureau: Japan Statistical Yearbook, 2: Population and Households.
http://www.stat.go.jp/english/data/nenkan/pdf/yhyou02.pdf
(Accessed 13 March 2017)

[3] Meng W, Liu Q, Zhou Z, Ai Q, Sheng B, Xie SS: Recent development of mechanisms and control strategies for robot-assisted lower limb rehabilitation.

47

Part 1

Mechatronics, Vol. 31, pp. 132-145, 2015.

DOI: 10.1016/j.mechatronics.2015.04.005

[4] Kita Y, Turin TC, Ichikawa M, Sugihara H, Morita Y, Tomioka N, Rumana N, Okayama A, Nakamura Y, Abbott RD, Ueshima H: Trend of stroke incidence in a Japanese population: Takashima stroke registry, 1990-2001. Int J Stroke, Vol. 4, pp. 241-249, 2009. DOI: 10.1111/j.1747-4949.2009.00293.x

[5] Sherrington C, Henschke N: Why does exercise reduce falls in older people? Unrecognised contributions to motor control and cognition? Br J Sports Med, Vol. 47, pp.731-732, 2013. DOI: 10.1136/bjsports-2012-091295

[6] TOYOTA: Toyota Robots Help People Walk Again: News Releases (28 May 2014). http://corporatenews.pressroom.toyota.com/releases/tmc+physical+rehabilitation+a id+robots+medical+facilities+may28.htm (Accessed 28 October 2016)

[7] HONDA: Honda Worldwide site: Walking Assist. http://world.honda.com/Walking-Assist/features/index.html (Accessed 28 October 2016)

[8] Taga G, Yamaguchi Y, Shimizu H: Self-organized control of bipedal locomotion by neural oscillators in unpredictable environment. Biol Cybern, Vol. 65, pp. 147-159, 1991.

[9] Yasuhara K, Shimada K, Koyama T, Ido T, Kickuchi K, Endo Y: Walking Assist Device with Stride Management System. Honda R&D Technical Review, Vol. 2, No. 2, 2009. https://www.hondarandd.jp/point.php?pid=122&lang=en (Accessed 28 October 2016)

[10] Buesing C, Fisch G, O'Donnell M, Shahidi I, Tomas L: Effects of wearable exoskeleton stride management assist system (SMA®) on spatiotemporal gait characteristics in individuals after stroke: a randomized controlled trial. J Neuroeng Rehabil, Vol. 12, P. 69, 2015. DOI: 10.1186/s12984-015-0062-0

[11] Shimada H, Suzuki T, Kimura Y, Hirata T, Sugiura M, Endo Y, Yasuhara K, Shimada K, Kikuchi K, Oda K, Ishii K, Ishiwata K: Effects of an automated stride assistance system on walking parameters and muscular glucose metabolism in

elderly adults. Br J Sports Med, Vol. 42, pp. 922-929, 2008. DOI: 10.1136/bjsm.2007.039453

[12] Ishihara K, Hirano S, Saitoh E, Tanabe S, Itoh N, Yanohara R, Katoh T, Sawada Y, Tsunoda T, Kagaya H: Characteristics of leg muscle activity in three different tasks using the balance exercise assist robot. Jpn J Compr Rehabil Sci, Vol. 6, pp. 105-112, 2015. DOI: 10.11336/jjcrs.6.105

[13] WIKIPEDIA: Inverted pendulum. https://en.wikipedia.org/wiki/Inverted_pendulum (Accessed 28 October 2016)

[14] Ozaki K, Kagaya H, Hirano S, Kondo I, Tanabe S, Itoh N, Saitoh E, Fuwa T, Murakami R: Preliminary trial of postural strategy training using a personal transport assistance robot for patients with central nervous system disorder. Arch Phys Med Rehabil, Vol. 94, pp. 59-66, 2013. DOI: 10.1016/j.apmr.2012.08.208

[15] Tanabe S, Saitoh E, Hirano S, Katoh M, Takemitsu T, Uno A, Shimizu Y, Muraoka Y, Suzuki T: Design of the Wearable Power-Assist Locomotor (WPAL) for paraplegic gait reconstruction. Disabil Rehabil Assist Technol, Vol. 8, pp. 84-91, 2013. DOI: 10.3109/17483107.2012.688238

[16] Tanabe S, Hirano S, Saitoh E: Wearable Power-Assist Locomotor (WPAL) for supporting upright walking in persons with paraplegia. Neurorehabilitation, Vol. 33, pp. 99-106, 2013. DOI: 10.3233/NRE-130932

[17] TOYOTA: Partner Robot Family. http://www.toyota-global.com/innovation/partner_robot/family_2.html (Accessed 28 October 2016)

[18] Ikeuchi Y, Ashihara J, Hiki Y, Kudoh H, Noda T: Walking assist device with bodyweight support system. Proceedings of 2009 IEEE International Conference on Intelligent Robots and Systems, 2009. DOI: 10.1109/IROS.2009.5354543

[19] HONDA: Honda Unveils Experimental Walking Assist Device with Bodyweight Support System. http://hondanews.com/releases/honda-unveils-experimental-walking-assist-device-with-bodyweight-support-system (Accessed 28 October 2016)

Part 1

[20] Bishop L, Stein J: Three upper limb robotic devices for stroke rehabilitation: A review and clinical perspective. Neurorehabilitation, Vol. 33, pp. 3-11, 2013. DOI: 10.3233/NRE-130922

Abstract

This chapter describes the methods to objectively evaluate the effectiveness of nursing care and nursing of the elderly with dementia. These methods will influence the efficiency of caring behaviors of robots and their effectiveness in demonstrating human care in nursing.

Key Words: Requisite performance, Nursing robots, Caring, Cooperation of engineers

Chapter IV

Evaluating the Effectiveness of Nursing Care Activities

for the Elderly with Dementia

By Yuko Yasuhara, Shoko Fuji, Hiroko Sugimoto, Kaori Kato

Part 1

1. Introduction

According to the Ministry of Internal Affairs and Communications, in 2015, the population of Japanese over 65 years old was 33.95 million, and accounted for 26.8% of the total population [1]. The total number of the elderly with dementia was about 4.63 million in 2012. Ninomiya, et al. are predicting that, based on the Hisayama study, the numbers of Japanese elderly persons with dementia will reach 6.75 million in 2025, if the prevalence of patients remains the same as that of 2012 [2]. The number of elderly with dementia and elderly persons who need intensive nursing care has also been increasing [3].

The primary symptoms of memory disorder and disorientation [4] among the elderly with dementia also show behavioral and psychological symptoms of dementia (BPSD) such as daytime drowsiness, nighttime delirium [5], and disturbed sleep [6-8]. It is possible that sleep disturbance alters life rhythms and affects the wandering behavior of the elderly, in addition to daytime drowsiness. It has been clarified that lack of sleep increases the risk for physiological dysfunctions such as those involving the autonomic nervous system [9, 10], endocrine system [11-16], or cardiovascular events [17-22].

Moreover, in Japan, caregiver burden has emerged as a social problem. This has been caused by the uniqueness of nuclear families, elderly care by the elderly wife, husband, or siblings [23]. This means there are not enough young people to take care of elderly people. From this situation, it is difficult for elderly caregivers to care for patients with dementia for a long period at home. Oftentimes, such patients live in long-term care facilities using their long-term care insurance benefits.

In 2015, the Ministry of Health, Labour and Welfare, launched the New Orange Plan [24] as the Japanese government's countermeasure program for the rapidly growing population of patients with dementia. Robotics for the elderly with dementia, and the promotion of research and development of models such as rehabilitation have been established. Furthermore, in 2014, with Japan's aging society and its falling childbirth rate, the government announced that "the New

52

Chapter IV

Robot Strategy" would be at work or implemented to help in robot development [25] as a possible answer to workforce demands. This is because nursing homes and long-term care health facilities have been faced with a chronic manpower shortage, and care robots such as communication robots have been found to be critical in this demanding role. In particular, it is necessary to consider the required function and performance of these nursing robots specific to the care of elderly patients with dementia.

Patients with long-term care insurances can receive rehabilitation services or recreational activities to maintain their "quality of life" in addition to treatments or nursing. The initial question that requires an appropriate and accurate answer is, "What kinds of functions are needed by robots to support the healthcare of elderly with dementia?" There are expectations that physiological changes caused by the care process will be clarified and robots that have effective functions will be developed to meet these demands for care.

This chapter describes the methods to evaluate effective nursing care for the elderly with dementia, and the availability of robots to improve elderly persons' autonomic nervous system and communication ability.

2. Method of objective evaluation

The following are published findings to clarify the daily activities, sleep condition, and autonomic nervous activity of the elderly with dementia [26] as compared to healthy persons. These findings explain the process of objective evaluations and characteristics using data derived from healthy persons and those of the elderly with dementia who reside at geriatric health services facility.

2.1. Measurement items
2.1.1. Actigraph
It is a measurement procedure that is used to assess the balance between waking time and sleeping time, and the conditions of sleep disturbance [27].

53

Part 1

Portable micro mini-type Actigraphs (Ambulatory Monitoring, Inc., Ardsley, NY, USA) were attached to each subject's non-dominant arm for 24 hours. It electronically measures the number of movements exceeding 0.01 g (gravitational force per minute of recording). An epoch length of 60 seconds was used from the vertical axis. The activity counts (AC) from the vertical axis of an accelerometer represent a digital integration of the positive and negative vertical displacement of the body's center of mass per unit time [28, 29]. Sleep or wake time was judged by the sleep-scoring algorithm of the AW2 software (Ambulatory Monitoring, Inc.) [30].

The time the subjects wore the Actigraph was divided into "waking time" intervals, defined as the period of time subjects reported being out of bed, and "sleeping time" intervals, defined as the period during which subjects were in bed. AC from the Actigraph were used as indicators of activity levels. The Actigraph was used in the zero crossing modes to detect a micro-motion.

2.1.2. Heart rate variability

Heart Rate Variability (HRV) is an efficient noninvasive method used to investigate autonomic nervous system function and cardiovascular control while awake or asleep. Electrodes were placed at strategic locations on the chest and recording was done via a Holter electrocardiographic monitor. This recording lasted for 24 hours. The low frequency (LF) component (0.04 - 0.15 Hz) is extracted by power spectrum density. The high frequency (HF) component (0.15 - 0.50 Hz) is extracted and serves as an indicator of parasympathetic nervous system activity. The LF/HF ratio indicates sympathetic nervous system activity.

2.1.3. Method of observing behaviors of subjects

Life records of the normal adults and elderly with dementia were shown along with the records taken by Actigraph and by HRV. In terms of the life records, activity details and the necessary times – the time when subjects went to bed, and the time when they woke up – were described on the autographic recording surveys.

54

Chapter IV

The healthy persons' activity statuses were further checked during the measurement period by interviewing them after the examination was over.

Methods of observing the elderly with dementia behaviors are as follows. During the daytime (9:00 - 17:00), four nurses who had more than five years' clinical experience observed the activities of the elderly with dementia while at nighttime (17:00 - 9:00), ten care workers cooperating with researchers who had more than five years' clinical experience replaced them. They recorded the activity status (including waking up, sleeping, and walking) of the elderly with dementia, along with their expressions and behaviors. During observation, the nurses and care workers maintained a certain distance from the subjects in case they should become too nervous.

These records were used to enhance the credibility of the analysis of the Actigraph and HRV results.

2.2. Statistical analysis

To clarify the relationship between autonomic nervous activity and AC, Pearson's correlation coefficient was calculated. The statistical analysis was carried out using the Statistical Package for the Social Sciences version 20 software (PASW Statistics for Windows, SPSS Inc., Chicago, IL, USA). Statistical significance was set at $p < 0.05$.

2.3. Diagnoses of dementia by HDS-R

The elderly with dementia were diagnosed using Hasegawa's Dementia Scale-Revised (HDS-R) [31]. With a HDS-R score of 20 or less, dementia was suspected (30 is the highest score possible). Other meanings of the HDS-R include severity of dementia: a score of 20 - 15 points is categorized as mild, 14 - 10 points is moderate, 9 - 5 points is moderately severe, and below 5 points is severe.

Long-term care levels (LTCL) classify the status of persons with problematic behavior and decreased understanding [32]. There are five levels. Level 1: Those who need some support for transfer movement; Level 2: Those who need some

Part 1

assistance for overall life; Level 3: Those who need greater assistance for transfer movement; Level 4: Those who cannot move or excrete by themselves; and Level 5: Those who cannot move, excrete, or eat by themselves.

3. Intensive communication with elderly with dementia is effective in maintaining their communication ability and daily life activity

Fig. 4-1 shows a typical example of normal 20's woman. Fig. 4-1 is unpublished data. Her AC in waking time was higher than during sleeping time. Sympathetic nerve activity also increased predominantly in waking time. Fig. 4-1 shows a negative correlation between HF and AC during awaking time (r = -0.400, p < 0.001), and positive correlation between LF/HF and AC during awaking time (r = 0.372, p < 0.001).

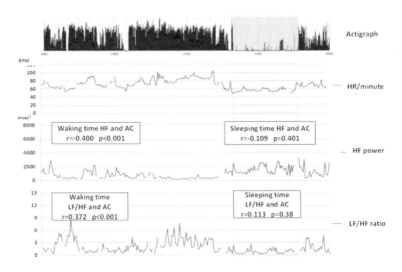

Fig. 4-1: Typical example of normal woman in her 20's with Actigraph and heart rate variability

Chapter IV

In healthy adults, parasympathetic nervous activity is predominant during sleep, whereas the sympathetic nervous system is active during waking time. There was a strong negative correlation between the AC and HF power, and a positive correlation between the AC and LF/HF ratio [33].

Fig. 4-2 and Fig. 4-3 are published [26]. Fig. 4-2 shows a typical example of Alzheimer's dementia in a woman in her early 80's who is LTCL 1 and has HDS-R 9 points (moderately severe). Her communication ability was good. She trained positively for recreation and rehabilitation. After lunch the subject took one tablet of Risperidone (0.5 mg) and one tablet of Diazepam (2 mg). This subject had the same autonomic nervous activity as a healthy person. It shows a positive correlation between LF/HF and AC ($r = 0.32$, $p < 0.001$), a negative correlation between HF and AC ($r = -0.25$, $p < 0.01$). During the day, she underwent rehabilitation for 62 minutes. The rehabilitation included upper and lower limb exercises and joint excursion training, as well as massage by an occupational therapist.

For the elderly with dementia as shown in Fig. 4-2, the suggestion is that physical activities and cognitive behavioral functions such as communication capabilities can be related to positive effects of sympathetic nervous activity [11].

57

Part 1

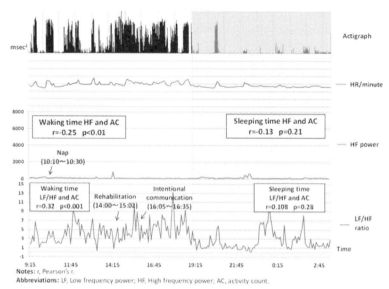

Fig. 4-2: Typical example of significant positive correlation between LF/HF and AC in the elderly with dementia during waking time

Fig. 4-3 shows a typical example of vascular dementia in a woman in her 60's who is LTCL 4 and has HDS-R 16 points (mild). She was using a wheelchair for movement; she required assistance transferring to the wheelchair. Her communication ability was not good; she can answer only Yes or No questions. She needs urging from care staff, but she regularly interrupts. Fig. 4-3 shows no correlation between LF/HF and AC ($r = 0.05$, $p = 0.512$), HF and AC ($r = -0.19$, $p < 0.05$) during sleeping and waking time, respectively. According to observation data, she was watching TV while in bed rest, and during the sleep period determined by Actigraph. However, her LF/HF did not change while watching TV, LH/FH and HF stayed at the same levels through 24 hours.

For the elderly with dementia as shown in Fig. 4-3, that shows low physical activities and low cognitive behavioral functions such as communication capabilities might not be able to change sympathetic nervous activity. It suggested that to have

Chapter IV

intensive communication with elderly with dementia is effective in maintaining their communication ability and daily life activity, and the necessity of strengthening the nursing care process that can maintain the communication ability and daily life activity of the elderly.

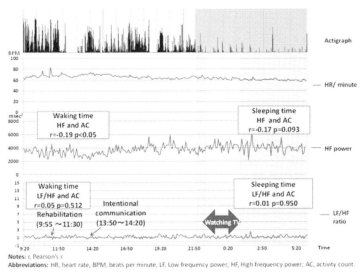

Fig. 4-3. Typical example of non-significant correlation between LF/HF and AC in the elderly with dementia during waking time

4. Can robots improve elderly persons' autonomic nervous system and communication abilities?

Initially, in the case of the elderly with dementia, they look like they have severely damaged cognitive functions and communication abilities. However, as indicated by the research findings, positive interpersonal exchange and physical activity are considered to provide effective autonomic nervous activity for them. Such nursing care practices maintain the patient's communication ability and daily

59

Part 1

life activity. It seems necessary to obtain more data to consider whether or not the robot can promote and improve an elderly person's autonomic nervous system and communication ability.

In Japan, "the New Robot Strategy" exists to develop technologies such as "helping" or assistive robots or human caring machines to compensate for the lack of caregivers. The use of robots with various technologies may possibly improve our human lives and, in particular, the lives of patients with dementia. Several robots have been developed with more sophisticated functions particularly for the elderly with dementia.

There are three types of robots concerned about elderly care, namely, the assistive robot, the entertainment robot, and the communication robot. The assistive robots have functions such as transfer [34], walking-aid [35], rehabilitation [36], excretion-assistance [37], and security. These robots can assist in the physical function of patients and care by the nurse. Humanoid robot "NAO [38]" and "PEPPER [39]" were developed by the Japanese branch office of Aldebaran Robotics Co., a subsidiary company of the Softbank Company. NAO has voice recognition software compatible with 19 languages. It can recognize such languages as the Kansai dialect in Japanese. PEPPER can also recognize the registered person's face, and can express emotions. The robot maintains constant conversation, and it can also store memories of events in its own data bank. Paro [40], a therapeutic robot baby harp seal, is intended to be very cute, to have a calming effect on the elderly, and then to evoke emotional responses similar to those in animal-assisted therapies.

It was considered that such robots provide healthy effects on the elderly persons' autonomic nervous activity and facilitate activities of daily living for the elderly with dementia. However, the effectiveness of such robots remain to be fully elucidated. To provide dependable effective results, it is necessary to objectively evaluate their effects more.

Chapter IV

5. Conclusion

As explained at the beginning of this chapter, some elderly with dementia are able to maintain communication skills, physical function, and autonomic nervous activity similar to healthy persons. It is anticipated that maintaining effective communication and physical activity might inhibit the progression of symptoms of dementia.

The care robots with communication abilities are being developed along the perspective of day to day activities. At some point in the near future, these care robots will be introduced in the clinical site. It will be important for human nurses to provide the optimal nursing care for their patients, otherwise, robots may replace them. Furthermore, it is important to clarify the role of human nurses in caring for elderly with dementia, and to address their respective roles in situations where humanoid robots may have become a dominant feature in healthcare settings.

References

[1] Ministry of Health, Labor and Welfare: Japan: About the Outlook for Japan's population composition.
http://www.mhlw.go.jp/seisakunitsuite/bunya/hukushi_kaigo/kaigo_koureisha/chiik i-houkatsu/dl/link1-1.pdf (in Japanese)

[2] Ministry of Health, Labor and Welfare: Japan: MHLY GRANTS SYSTEM, National Institute of Public, Health.
https://mhlw-grants.niph.go.jp/niph/search/NIDD00.do?resrchNum=201405037A (in Japanese) (Accessed 6 September 2016)

[3] Ministry of Health, Labor and Welfare: Japan: About the Current State of Nursing Care Facilities, 2015

[4] American Psychiatric Association. Diagnostic and Statistical Manual of Mental Disorders, Fifth Edition (DSM-5), American Psychiatric Association, Arlington, 2013.

[5] Elie M, Cole M, Primeau F, et al.: Delirium risk factors in elderly hospitalized patients. J Gen Intern Med, Vol.13, pp. 204-312, 1998.

[6] Rongve A, Boeve BF, Aarsland D: Frequency and correlates of caregiver-reported sleep disturbances in a sample of persons with early dementia. J Am Geriatr Soc, Vol. 58, pp. 480-486, 2010.

[7] Cerejeira J, Lagarto L, Mukaetova-Ladinska EB: Behavioral and Psychological Symptoms of Dementia. Front Neurol. Vol. 73, No. 3, 2012. (DOI:10.3389/fneur.2012.00073)

[8] Mishima K, Tozawa T, Satoh K, et al.: Melatonin secretion rhythm disorders in patients with senile dementia of Alzheimer's type with disturbed sleep-waking. Biol Psychiatry, Vol. 45, No. 4, pp. 417-421, 1999.

[9] Tochikubo O, Ikeda A, Miyajima E, et al.: Effects of insufficient sleep on blood pressure monitored by a new multibiomedical recorder. Hypertension, Vol. 27, pp. 1318-1324, 1996.

[10] Spiegel K, Leproult R, Van CE: Impact of sleep debt on metabolic and endocrine function. Lancet. Vol. 354, pp. 1435-1439, 1999.

[11] Beihl DA, Liese AD, Haffner SM: Sleep duration as a risk factor for incident type 2 diabetes in a multiethnic cohort. Ann Epidemiol, Vol. 19, pp. 351-357, 2009.

[12] Chaput JP, Despres JP, Bouchard C, Astrup A, et al.: Sleep duration as a risk factor for the development of type 2 diabetes or impaired glucose tolerance: analyses of the Quebec Family Study. Sleep Med, Vol. 10, pp. 919-924, 2009.

[13] Gangwisch JE, Heymsfield SB, Boden-Albala B, Buijs RM, Kreier F, Pickering TG, Rundle AG, Zammit GK, Malaspina D: Sleep duration as a risk factor for diabetes incidence in a large US sample. Sleep, Vol. 30, pp. 1667-1673, 2007.

[14] Mallon L, Broman J, Hetta J: High incidence of diabetes in men with sleep complaints or short sleep duration: a 12-year follow-up study of a middle-aged population. Diabetes Care, Vol. 28, pp. 2762-2767, 2005.

[15] Xu Q, Song Y, Hollenbeck A, Blair A, Schatzkin A, Chen H: Day napping and short night sleeping are associated with higher risk of diabetes in older adults. Diabetes Care, Vol. 33, pp. 78-83, 2010.

Chapter IV

[16] Gottlieb DJ, Punjabi NM, Newman AB, Resnick HE, Redline S, Baldwin CM, Nieto FJ: Association of sleep time with diabetes mellitus and impaired glucose tolerance. Arch Intern Med, Vol. 165, pp. 863-867, 2005.

[17] Amagai Y, Ishikawa S, Gotoh T, Kayaba K, Nakamura Y, Kajii E: Sleep duration and incidence of cardiovascular events in a Japanese population: the Jichi Medical School cohort study. J Epidemiol, Vol. 20, pp. 106-110, 2010.

[18] Ayas NT, White DP, Manson JE, Stampfer MJ, Speizer FE, Malhotra A, Hu FB: A prospective study of sleep duration and coronary heart disease in women. Arch Intern Med, Vol. 163, pp. 205-209, 2003.

[19] Burazeri G, Gofin J, Kark JD: Over 8 hours of sleep-marker of increased mortality in Mediterranean population: follow-up population study. Croat Med J, Vol. 44, pp. 193-198, 2003.

[20] Hamazaki Y , Morikawa Y , Nakamura K, Sakurai M, Miura K, Ishizaki M, Kido T, Naruse Y , Suwazono Y , Nakagawa H: The effects of sleep duration on the incidence of cardiovascular events among middle-aged male workers in Japan. Scand J Work Environ Health, Vol.37, pp. 411-417, 2011.

[21] Meisinger C, Heier M, Lowel H, Schneider A, Doring A: Sleep duration and sleep complaints and risk of myocardial infarction in middle-aged men and women from the general population: The MONICA/KORA Augsburg cohort study. Sleep, Vol. 69, No. 30, pp. 1121-1127, 2007.

[22] Shankar A, Koh WP, Yuan JM, Lee HP, Yu M: Sleep Duration and Coronary Heart Disease Mortality Among Chinese Adults in Singapore: A Population-based Cohort Study. Am J Epidemiol, Vol. 168, pp. 1367-1373, 2008.

[23] Miyamoto Y, Tachimori H, Ito H: Formal caregiver burden in dementia: impact of behavioral and psychological symptoms of dementia and activities of daily living. Geriatr Nurs, Vol. 31, No. 4, pp. 246-532, 2010.

[24] Ministry of Health, Labour and Welfare: Japan: New Orange Plan. http://www.mhlw.go.jp/stf/seisakunitsuite/bunya/0000064084.html (in Japanese) (Accessed 6 September 2016)

Part 1

[25] Japan: Ministry of Economy, Trade and Industry, Japan's robot strategy, http://www.meti.go.jp/press/2014/01/20150123004/20150123004b.pdf (in Japanese)

[26] Fuji S, Tanioka T, Yasuhara Y, Sato M, Saito K, Purnell MJ, Locsin RC, Yasui T: Characteristic Autonomic Nervous Activity of Institutionalized Elders with Dementia, Open Journal of Psychiatry, Vol. 6, pp. 34-49, 2016.

[27] Chung GS, Choi BH, Jeong DU, Park KS: Noninvasive Heart Rate Variability Analysis Using Load cell -Installed Bed during Sleep. Proceedings of the 29th Annual International Conference of the IEEE EMBS, Lyon, 22-26 August 2007, pp.2357-2360, 2007.

[28] Sandroff BM, Motl RW, Suh Y: Accelerometer Output and Its Association with Energy Expenditure in Persons with Multiple Sclerosis. Journal of Rehabilitation Research & Development, Vol. 49, pp. 467-476, 2012.
DOI: 10.1682/JRRD.2011.03.0063

[29] Hjorth MF, Chaput JP, Michaelsen K, Astrup A, Tetens I, Sjödin A: Seasonal Variation in Objectively Measured Physical Activity, Sedentary Time, Cardio-Respiratory Fitness and Sleep Duration among 8-11 Year Old Danish Children: A Repeated-Measures Study. BMC Public Health, Vol. 13, p. 808, 2013.
DOI: 10.1186/1471-2458-13-808

[30] Cole RJ, Kripke DF, Gruen W, Mullaney DJ, Gillin JC: Automatic Sleep/Wake Identification from Wrist Activity. Sleep, Vol. 15, pp. 461-469, 1992.

[31] Imai Y, Hasegawa K: The Revised Hasegawa's Dementia Scale (HDS-R) – Evaluation of Its Usefulness Screening Test for Dementia. Hong Kong Journal of Psychiatry, Vol. 4, pp. 20-24, 1994.

[32] Ministry of Health, Labor and Welfare: Japan: The Long-Term Care Insurance System. http://www.mhlw.go.jp/english/topics/elderly/care/2.html

[33] Satoh M, Yasuhara Y, Tanioka T, Iwasa Y, Miyake M, Yasui T, Tomotake M, Kobayashi H, Locsin RC: Measuring quality of sleep and autonomic nervous function in healthy Japanese women, Neuropsychiatric Disease and Treatment, Vol. 2014, No. 10, pp. 89-96, 2014.

Chapter IV

[34] RIKEN, Japan. http://www.riken.jp/en/pr/press/2015/20150223_2/

[35] Honda Motor Co. http://world.honda.com/HondaRobotics/index.html

[36] Cyberdyne Inc.: What is HAAL® (Hybrid Assistive Limb®).
http://www.cyberdyne.jp/english/products/HAL/

[37] Daiwa House Industry Co.: About the Minelet.
http://www.daiwahouse.co.jp/robot/minelet/contact.html (in Japanese)

[38] PC watch HP. http://pc.watch.impress.co.jp/docs/news/20140618_653931.html

[39] SoftBank group HP: Alswbaran. https://www.aldebaran.com/en/cool-robots/pepper

[40] FUJISOFT Inc. HP: PALRO is a robot who cares. https://palro.jp/en/

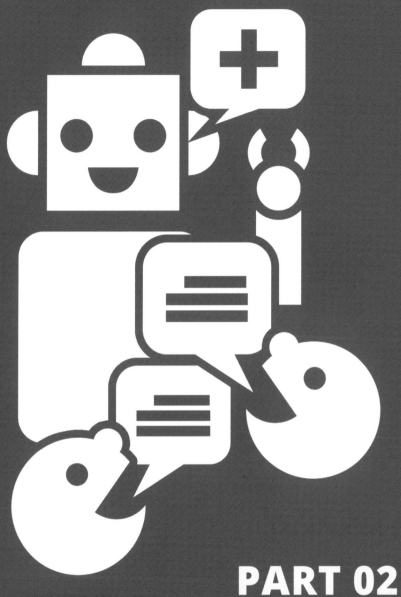

PART 02

The communication capabilities required for humanoid nursing robots, and for the future of robot care in 2050.

© 2017 Illustrated by Leo Vicente Bollos

Part 2

Abstract

This chapter introduces the history, definition, and the basic components of robots. Also discussed are the safety of robots and explanation of the safety measures of robots in both Japan and overseas.

Key Words: Robot, History and definition of robots, Basic components of robots, Safety of robots

---

Chapter V

What are Robots?

By Yoshihiro Kai

Chapter V

1. Introduction

In many countries, the number of elderly persons is rapidly increasing, especially in Japan [1, 2]. Human-friendly robots which support humans within human environments such as Nursing Robots will be needed more and more in the very near future. Many researchers have developed human-friendly robots [3-10]. However, robotics is a relatively young research field.

As presented in this chapter, the history of robots is relatively short. In order for human-friendly robots such as nursing robots to be widely used in the future, many issues such as the development of laws, insurance institutes, etc. need to be addressed and explained. In the technological field, improving the safety of the robots is one of the future issues.

In this chapter, the history and definition of robots are introduced, including the basic components of robots. Furthermore, the safety of robots and the safety measures instituted are discussed and explained.

2. The history of robots

The word "Robot" is derived from the Czech word "robota" which was used in a 1921 play Rossum's Universal Robots (R.U.R.) by the Czech writer, Karel Čapek (1890-1938) [11]. The word "robota" means "servitude" or "forced labor". Robots originally existed in imaginary worlds.

In 1954, George Devol (1912-2011) applied for a patent for the first robot in the real world [12]. Joseph Frederick Engelberger (1925-2015) and Devol formed the world's first robot manufacturing company, Unimation. The first industrial robot, Unimate, was mainly used to transfer objects from one point to another in an industrial plant. Therefore, it was also called "Programmed article transfer". After that, various kinds of industrial robots were developed and produced to work in industrial plants such as automobile plants.

69

Part 2

Recently, many robots have been developed to work in human environments as well. The communication robot "Parlo" (FUJI SOFT INCORPORATED) [13], the robotic vacuum cleaner "Roomba" (iRobot Corporation) [14], the humanoid robot "Asimo" (Honda Motor Co., Ltd.) [15], the robot suit "HAL" (CYBERDYNE Inc.) [16], and the autonomous hospital delivery robot "HOSPI" (Panasonic Corporation) [17], are examples, to name a few.

3. The definition of robots

International Organization for Standardization (ISO) 8373 (Robots and robotic devices – Vocabulary) second edition defines robots as the following [18]:

Actuated mechanism programmable in two or more axes with a degree of autonomy, moving within its environment, to perform intended tasks; a robot includes the control system and interface of the control system; the classification of robot into industrial robot or service robot is done according to its intended application.

Industrial robots are defined as the following:

Automatically controlled, re-programmable, multipurpose manipulator, programmable in three or more axes, which can be either fixed in place or mobile for use in industrial automation applications.

Furthermore, service robots are defined as the following:

Robot that performs useful tasks for humans or equipment excluding industrial automation applications.

Robots including service robots had never been defined before the ISO 8373 second edition appeared in 2012. Only industrial robots are defined in ISO 8373 first edition [19]. Therefore, the definition of robots may change over time.

70

Chapter V

4. The basic components of robots

In order to perform the functions indicated in the aforementioned definitions, robots are generally equipped with sensors, controllers (including computers), and actuators. The controllers control the actuators based on the information measured by the sensors. Robot arms, legs, and wheels, etc. are driven by the actuators.

4.1. Sensor

Sensors used for robots are divided into the following two types (Fig. 5-1):

(1) Internal state sensor

This sensor measures the internal state of a robot (e.g. Joint angle).

For example, potentiometer, encoder, accelerometer, etc.

(2) External state sensor

This sensor measures the external state of a robot (e.g. the distance between the robot and an object, the contact force between the robot and an object, etc.).

For example, Distance sensor, Camera, Global Positioning System (GPS), Force sensor, Tactile sensor, etc.

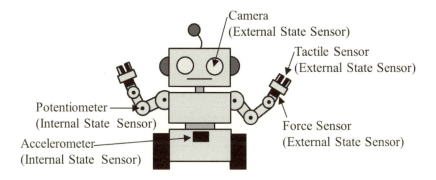

Fig. 5-1: Sensors used for robots

71

Part 2

4.2. Actuator

Actuators are power mechanisms for moving robots. Electrical actuators (generally called motors), hydraulic actuators, and pneumatic actuators are mainly used as robotic actuators.

5. The safety of robots

In order for human-friendly robots such as nursing robots to enjoy wide use in the future, it is important to improve their safety features [20]. In industrial robots, the safety of humans is guaranteed by isolating the robots from humans. However, it is difficult to isolate human-friendly robots from humans because the robots work within human environments. Therefore, many safety measures have been proposed as shown below.

5.1. Emergency switch

Emergency switches are generally used as robots' safety devices [21-23]. When emergency switches are pushed, the robot stops.

5.2. Low power motors

We can use low power motors so as not to injure humans in collisions between the robot and humans [24].

5.3. Shock absorbing materials and/or passive compliant joint mechanisms

In order to reduce the impact force in collisions between the robot and humans, shock absorbing materials [25, 26] and/or passive compliant joint mechanisms [27, 28] are used.

Chapter V

5.4. Safety measure using a computer

When a robot's computer operates functionally, it uses sensor signals to detect unexpected motions and then, once these motions are detected, to stop the robot.

5.5. Safety measure using electrical switches/sensors

Electrical switches/sensors (e.g. proximity switches [29], tactile sensors [30], etc.) are often used to detect unexpected robot motions and switch off all the robot's motors.

5.6. Safety measure using power-off holding brakes

We can use the electrical switches/sensors shown in 5.5 in order to guarantee safety even when the robot's computer breaks down. However, if the robot is on a slope and its batteries die, it will pose a hazard because the robot will move down the slope at a high speed with gravity (Fig. 5-2(a)). Also, the robot may still collide with humans due to the inertial force even after the switches/sensors switch off the motors. Power-off holding brakes are used to stop the robot when its batteries die on a slope [31]. When there is no power, the power-off holding brakes are automatically activated and they stop the robot (Fig. 5-2(b)). However, if a robot presses a human against a wall after the batteries die or the power is disconnected by an emergency switch, it will be difficult to rescue the human because the brakes are activated.

73

Part 2

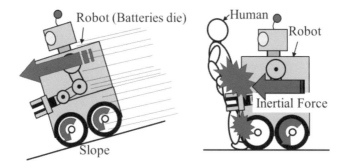

(a) Without electromagnetic brakes

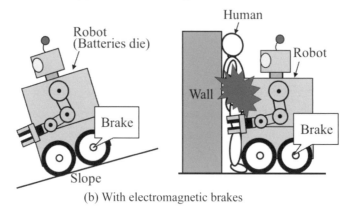

(b) With electromagnetic brakes

Fig. 5-2: Safety issues

5.7. ER/MR clutches

Electrorheological clutches (ER clutches) [32] and/or magnetorheological clutches (MR clutches) [33] can cut off the torque transmissions to the robot's joints by using a computer. In order not to exert unexpected high torques on robot's joints, we can use ER clutches and/or MR clutches. However, they may not be able to cut off the torque transmissions when the computer breaks down. Moreover, they require a power supply.

Chapter V

5.8. Joint limiter

Joint limiters are often used in exoskeleton robots, etc. [34]. Joint limiters are useful in order to prevent hyperextension of human joints when the robot's computer does not operate functionally.

5.9. Velocity, torque, and contact force-based mechanical safety devices for wheeled mobile robots

Safety is one of the most important issues in human-friendly robots which support humans within human environments. Human safety should be guaranteed even when the robot's computer breaks down.

The emergency switches introduced in 5.1. are useful for stopping the robot when the robot's computer does not work. However, humans may not be able to push the emergency switch in case of an emergency. As for the low power motors introduced in 5.2., the robots using these motors may not be able to perform given tasks. Furthermore, preventing the robot from colliding with humans at high speeds or exerting a large force on humans is still more desirable even when we can rely on the shock absorbing materials and/or the passive compliant joint mechanisms shown in 5.3.

When we use the electrical switches/sensors, the power-off holding brakes, or ER/MR clutches, the problems shown in 5.6. and 5.7. present themselves.

5.9.1. Velocity-based mechanical safety device for wheeled mobile robots

The "velocity-based mechanical safety device for wheeled mobile robots" was developed to address the above problems [35]. The safety device consists of only mechanical passive components without actuators, controllers, or batteries. The safety device is attached to each of the robot's drive-shafts. The features of the velocity-based safety device are as follows:

(i) If the angular velocity of a drive-shaft exceeds a preset threshold level in one direction, then the safety device switches off all the robot's motors and

75

Part 2

locks the drive-shaft in that direction. The preset threshold level is called the "detection velocity level". We expect the safety device to prevent the robot from colliding with humans at unexpected high speeds (Fig. 5-3(a)).

(ii) The detection velocity level is adjustable. We can set the detection velocity level after taking each task into consideration.

(iii) The drive-shaft is unlocked by rotating it in the opposite direction where it was locked. So, if a robot locked by the safety device presses a human against a wall, we can easily rescue the human by moving the robot in the opposite direction in which the human is being held (Fig. 5-3(b)).

(iv) The safety device consists of only passive components without actuators, controllers, or batteries. Even after the batteries in the robot have died, the safety device works because it requires no power supply (Fig. 5-3(c)).

Chapter V

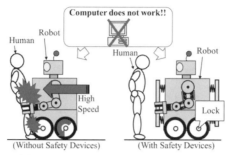
(a) Unexpected high speed robot motion

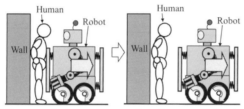
(b) Rescue of a human pressed against a wall by the robot

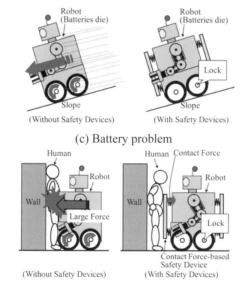
(c) Battery problem

(d) Low speed robot motion after the controller has broken down

Fig. 5-3: Mechanical safety devices

77

Part 2

5.9.2. Torque-based mechanical safety device for wheeled mobile robots

The velocity-based mechanical safety devices cannot stop the robot if the unexpected high velocity does not occur in each drive-shaft when the robot's computer breaks down. Both the velocity-based mechanical safety devices and the "torque-based mechanical safety devices" should be used to further assure human safety [36]. A torque limiter [37] and a switch are used in the torque-based mechanical safety device. The torque-based safety device is also attached to each of the robot's drive-shafts. The features of the torque-based safety device are as follows:

(i) If the torque of a drive-shaft exceeds a preset threshold level, then the safety device for the drive-shaft cuts off the torque transmission and switches off all the robot's motors. The preset threshold level is called the "detection torque level".

(ii) The detection torque level is adjustable.

(iii) The safety device consists of only passive components without actuators, controllers, or batteries.

With the first and third feature, we expect the safety device to prevent the robot from exerting an unexpected large force on humans – if the angular velocity of each drive-shaft does not exceed the detection velocity level when the computer breaks down. Furthermore, the second feature allows us to adjust the detection torque level after taking each task into consideration.

5.9.3. Contact force-based mechanical safety device for wheeled mobile robots

If the detection torque level is set too low in the above torque-based safety device, the robot may not be able to go up a slope. On the other hand, if the detection torque level is set too high, the robot may exert a large force on humans.

The "contact force-based mechanical safety device" was developed to solve this problem [38, 39]. As shown in Figure 5-3(d), the contact force-based safety

Chapter V

devices are attached on the robot's outer surfaces. The features of the contact force-based safety device are as follows:

(i) If the contact force acting on a contact force-based safety device exceeds a threshold level, then the safety device switches off all the robot's motors and locks the drive-shaft in the opposite direction of the contact force (Fig. 5-3(d)). The threshold level is called the "detection contact force level".

(ii) The drive-shaft is unlocked by rotating it in the opposite direction where it was locked.

(iii) The safety device consists of only passive components without actuators, controllers, or batteries.

With the first and third features, we expect the safety device to prevent the robot from exerting an unexpected large force on humans – if the angular velocity of each drive-shaft does not exceed the detection velocity level when the controller breaks down (Fig. 5-3(d)). If a human is pressed against a wall by the robot locked by the safety device, the second feature allows us to rescue the human easily by moving the robot in the opposite direction where the human is being held (Fig. 5-3(b)).

5.10. Velocity and torque-based mechanical safety devices for exoskeleton robots

We can expect exoskeleton robots to be applied in many fields. However, safety is one of the most important issues in exoskeleton robots. Exoskeleton robots with hardware-based safety devices are needed to guarantee safety even when the computers do not operate functionally.

Emergency switches or joint limiters are often used in hardware-based safety devices. However, humans may not be able to push the emergency switch in case of an emergency. Furthermore, joint limiters involve risks such as (1) the exoskeleton robot moving a human leg at an unexpected high velocity (Fig. 5-4(a)), and (2) exerting unexpected high torques on human joints (Fig. 5-4(b)), before the joint limiters can stop the exertion.

79

Part 2

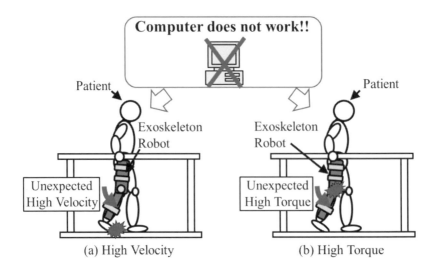

Fig. 5-4: Problem in the case of computer failure

Two hardware-based safety devices – the "velocity-based safety device" and the "torque-based safety device" have been developed to address this problem [40-43].

The features of the velocity-based safety device are as follows:
(i) If the angular velocity of the motor exceeds a preset threshold level, then the safety device switches off the motor. The preset threshold level is called the "detection velocity level". We expect the velocity-based safety device to prevent the exoskeleton robot from forcing the human leg to move at high speeds.
(ii) The detection velocity level is adjustable. We can adjust the detection velocity level after taking each task into consideration.

Also, the features of the torque-based safety device are as follows:
(i) If the torque the exoskeleton robot exerts on a human joint exceeds a preset threshold level, then the safety device switches off the motor. The preset

Chapter V

threshold level is called the "detection torque level". We expect the torque-based safety device to prevent the exoskeleton robot from exerting an unexpected high torque on the human.

(ii) The detection torque level is adjustable. We can adjust the detection torque level after taking each task into consideration.

6. Conclusion

In this chapter, we explained the history of robots. Next, we described the definition of robots and indicated that the definition of robots will change over time. Thirdly, we explained the basic components of robots. Finally, we described that the safety of robots is one of the most important issues in human-friendly robots and explained the safety measures of robots in both Japan and overseas.

Robotics engineers should make efforts to develop 100% safe robots. However, it will be impossible to develop such perfectly safe robots. Therefore, users should understand that 100% safe robots do not exist and use the robots carefully.

In order for human-friendly robots to enjoy wide use in the future, it will be necessary to improve not only the safety but also the communication ability of robots.

References

[1]   United Nations Population Fund (UNFPA) and Help Age International, Ageing in the Twenty-First Century: A Celebration and A Challenge. United Nations Population Fund and Help Age International, pp. 19-26, 2013.

[2]   Cabinet Office, Government of Japan: Annual Report on the Aging Society: 2015 (Summary). Cabinet Office Japan, pp. 2-8, 2015.

[3]   Tani T, Koseki A, Sakai A, Hattori S, Ouchi A: System design and field-testing of the walking training system. Proceedings of 1996 IEEE/RSJ International Conference on Intelligent Robots and Systems, Vol. 1, pp. 340-345, 1996.

Part 2

[4] Tanioka T, Kai Y, Matsuda T, Inoue Y, Sugawara K, Takasaka Y, Tsubahara A, Matsushita Y, Nagamine I, Tada T, Hashimoto F: Real-time measurement of frozen gait in patient with parkinsonism using a sensor-controlled walker. The Journal of Medical Investigation, Vol. 51, pp. 108-116, 2004.

[5] Mukai T, Hirano S, Nakashima H, Kato Y, Sakaida Y, Guo S, Hosoe S: Development of a Nursing-Care Assistant Robot RIBA That Can Lift a Human in Its Arms. Proceedings of 2010 IEEE/RSJ International Conference on Intelligent Robots and Systems, pp. 5996-6001, 2010.

[6] Miyawaki K, Iwami T, Obinata G, Kondo Y, Kutsuzawa K, Ogasawara Y, Nishimura S: Evaluation of the gait for elderly people using an assisting cart (Gait on flat surface). JSME Int. J, Series C, Vol. 43, No. 4, pp. 966-974, 2000.

[7] Lee J, Lee C: Development of Walking Assistance Robot System and Experiment with the Disabled. Proceedings of SICE/ICASE Workshop, pp. 219-224, 2001.

[8] Kaneko K, Kanehiro F, Morisawa M, Akachi K, Miyamori G, Hayashi A, Kanehira N, Miyamori G, Hayashi A, Kanehira N: Humanoid Robot HRP-4 – Humanoid Robotics Platform with Lightweight and Slim Body –. Proceedings of 2011 IEEE/RSJ International Conference on Intelligent Robots and Systems, pp. 4400-4407, 2011.

[9] Iwata H, Sugano S: Design of human symbiotic robot TWENDY-ONE. Proceedings of 2009 IEEE International Conference on Robotics and Automation, pp. 580-586, 2009.

[10] Seto F, Kosuge K, Hirata Y: Self-collision avoidance motion control for human robot cooperation system using RoBE. Proceedings of 2005 IEEE/RSJ International Conference on Intelligent Robots and Systems, pp.3143-3148, 2005.

[11] Yoneda K, Tsubouchi T, Ohkuma H: The first robot creation design. Koudansya Scientific, 2003. (in Japanese)

[12] Masuda R, Koganezawa K, Kai Y: New Robot Engineering. Shokodo Co., LTD., 2006. (in Japanese)

Chapter V

[13] FUJI SOFT INCORPORATED. http://www.fsi.co.jp/e/index.html

[14] iRobot: Roomba Robot Vacuum.

https://www.irobot.com/For-the-Home/Vacuuming/Roomba.aspx

[15] Honda Worldwide: Honda Robotics. http://world.honda.com/HondaRobotics/

[16] CYBERDYNE: The world's first cyborg-type robot "HAL®".

http://www.cyberdyne.jp/products/HAL/

[17] Panasonic: HOSPi. http://www.panasonic.com/jp/company/ppe/hospi.html

[18] ISO 8373 Second Edition: Robots and robotic devices – Vocabulary, 2012.

[19] ISO 8373 First Edition: Manipulating industrial robots – Vocabulary, 1994.

[20] ISO 13482 First Edition: Robots and robotic devices – Safety requirements for personal care robots, 2014.

[21] Nemoto Y, Egawa S, Koseki A, Hattori S, Ishii T, Fujie M: Power assisted Walking Support System for Elderly. proceedings of the 20th Annual International Conference of the IEEE Eng. in Medicine and Biology Soc., Vol. 20, No. 5, pp. 2693-2695, 1998.

[22] Kai Y, Tanioka T, Inoue Y, Matsuda T, Sugawara K, Takasaka Y, Nagamine I: A Walking Support/Evaluation Machine for Patients with Parkinsonism. The Journal of Medical Investigation, Vol. 51, pp. 117-124, 2004.

[23] Kawamoto H, Lee S, Kanbe S, Sankai Y: Power assist method for HAL-3 using EMG-based feedback controller. Proceedings of International Conference on Systems, Man and Cybernetics (SMC2003), pp. 1648-1653, 2003.

[24] Fukase A: Safety measures of meal-assistance robot – my spoon –. Journal of the Robotics Society of Japan, Vol. 25, No. 8, pp. 1165-1167, 2007. (in Japanese)

[25] Suita K, Yamada Y, Tsuchida N, Imai K, Ikeda H, Sugimoto N: A failure-to-safety "Kyozon" system with simple contact detection and stop capabilities for safe human-autonomous robot coexistence. Proceedings of IEEE International Conference on Robotics and Automation, pp. 3089-3096, 1995.

[26] Sugaiwa T, Iwata H, Sugano S: Shock absorbing skin design for human-symbiotic robot at the worst case collision. Proceedings of 2008 IEEE-RAS International Conference on Humanoid Robots, pp.481-486, 2008.

83

Part 2

[27] Yoon SS, Kang S, Kim SJ, Kim YH, Kim M, Lee CW: Safe arm with MR-based passive compliant joints and visco-elastic covering for service robot applications. Proceedings of 2003 IEEE/RSJ International Conference on Intelligent Robots and Systems, pp. 2191-2196, 2003.

[28] Koganezawa K, Shimizu Y, Inomata H, Nakazawa T: Actuator with non Linear elastic system (ANLES) for controlling joint stiffness on antaonistic driving. Proceedings of 2004 IEEE International Conference on Robotics and Biomimetics, pp. 51-55, 2004.

[29] Azbil Corp.: Environment-resistant switch. 2012. http://www.azbil.com/products/factory/download/catalog-spec/CP-PC-2256E-00.pdf

[30] Elkmann N, Fritzsche M, Schulenburg E: Tactile sensing for safe physical human-robot interaction. Proceedings of 4th International Conference on Advances in Computer-Human Interactions, pp. 212-217, 2011.

[31] Yasukawa electric corporation: "AC Servomotor SAFETY PRECAUTIONS", 2009.

[32] Sakaguchi M, Zhang G, Furusho J: Modeling and motion control of an actuator unit using ER clutches. Proceedings of IEEE International Conference on Robotics and Automation, San Francisco, pp. 1347-1353, 2000.

[33] Takesue N, Asaoka H, Lin J, Sakaguchi M, Zhang G, Furusho J: Development and experiments of actuator using MR fluid. Proceedings of 26th Annual Conference of the IEEE Industrial Electronics Society, pp. 1838-1843, 2000.

[34] Chen F, Yu Y, Ge Y, Sun J, Deng X: A PAWL for enhancing strength and endurance during walking using interaction force and dynamical information. Climbing and Walking Robots: towards New Applications, pp. 417-428, 2007.

[35] Kai Y: Development of a walking support robot with velocity-based mechanical safety devices. Proceedings of 2013 IEEE/RSJ International Conference on Intelligent Robots and Systems, pp. 1125-1130, 2013.

[36] Kai Y, Arihara K, Kitaguchi S: Development of a walking support robot with velocity and torque-based mechanical safety devices. Proceedings of 2014 IEEE

Chapter V

International Conference on Advanced Intelligent Mechatronics, pp. 1498-1503, 2014.

[37] Tsubakimoto Chain Co.: Tsubaki SAFCON overload protection and control devices. pp. 15-19, 2013.

[38] Kai Y, Sando S: Development of a Velocity and Contact Force-based Mechanical Safety Device for Service Robots. Proceedings of 2014 IEEE International Conference on Automation Science and Engineering, pp. 1188-1193, 2014.

[39] Kai Y, Arihara K: A Walking Support Robot with Velocity, Torque, and Contact Force-based Mechanical Safety Devices. Proceedings of 2015 IEEE/RSJ International Conference on Intelligent Robots and Systems, pp. 5026-5031, 2015.

[40] Kai Y, Kitaguchi S, Zhang W, Tomizuka M: Design of a rehabilitation robot suit with hardware-based safety devices - Proposal of the basic structure -. Proceedings of the Eighteenth International Symposium on Artificial Life and Robotics 2013, pp. 585-588, 2013.

[41] Kai Y, Kitaguchi S, Kanno S, Zhang W, Tomizuka M: Development of a Rehabilitation Robot Suit with Velocity and Torque-based Mechanical Safety Devices. Proceedings of 2014 IEEE/RSJ International Conference on Intelligent Robots and Systems, pp. 1380-1385, 2014.

[42] Kai Y, Kanno S, Zhang W, Tomizuka M: A Robot Suit with Hardware-based Safety Devices: Frequency Response Analysis of a Velocity-based Safety Device. Proceedings of 2015 IEEE/ASME International Conference on Advanced Intelligent Mechatronics, pp. 641-646, 2015.

[43] Noguchi S, Kai Y, Tomizuka M: A Robot Suit with Hardware-based Safety Devices: Transient Response Analysis of a Velocity-based Safety Device. Proceedings of 2015 IEEE/SICE International Symposium on System Integration, pp. 253-258, 2015.

85

Part 2

Abstract

This chapter describes empathic understanding in human-robot communication that has become an essential factor in the development of humanoid nurse robots (HNRs). The establishments of critical parameters toward advancing the technological competency of the HNRs within the certainties of the human nurse-caring perspective are expected. Empathic understanding provides the incentive to design and develop human nurses, HNRs, and human caring technologies from a caring science perspective.

Key Words: Empathic understanding, Nursing, Nurse-robot, Communication, Caring

---

Chapter VI

Empathic Understanding in Human-Robot

Communication: Influences on Caring in Nursing

By Kyoko Osaka

Chapter VI

1. Introduction

Communication between patients and nurses is a core activity of nursing care. The American Association of Critical Care Nurses emphasized that "Nurses must be as proficient in communication skills as they are in clinical skills" [1]. Initiating the development of skilled communication must include: (1) understanding the importance of a climate of safety; (2) acknowledging one's mental status; and (3) realizing that the only people we control are ourselves [2]. In communication, "empathy" is a term that is often heard, particularly in nursing practice.

Empathy appears to have its origin in the German word "Einfulung" which means "feeling within" [3, 4]. Empathy is one of the significant topics internalized by a nurse if he/her is to practice nursing well. Nevertheless, some take it for granted that caring and compassion, empathy and sympathy are inclusive and often interchangeable terms in nursing [5] making empathy an elusive concept [6].

Rogers [7], a psychologist, used the term "empathic understanding" to describe the caring skill of temporarily laying aside our views and values for entering into another's world without prejudice. The empathic understanding of the client's intentional frame of reference is an attempt to attend to the whole person (not only the person's feelings) by trying to absorb and respond to the person's view of his/her world including his/her various reactions and feelings. This concept includes the view that reciprocal relationships develop between nurses and patients during the course of nursing care. It is critical therefore that a reciprocal relationship between humans and robots and trustworthy relationship among nurses, humanoid nurse robots (HNRs), and patients exist during the course of nursing care.

The technology in communications between humans and robots has advanced exponentially. Robotics research on emotions and empathy is one of the most active domains of contemporary science, in which robot communication research have increased dramatically since the beginning of the first half of the 20th century.

Human communication includes not only verbal exchange but also facial expressions, gestures, and other nonverbal communication processes. Researchers

87

Part 2

have been interested in equipping robots with communication functions that enable robots to behave and respond realistically like a human being.

Verbal communication in robots needs to include voice recognition, language understanding, dialogue management, response generation, and voice synthesis. These are some of the essential processes of robot communication. Furthermore, expression recognition and motion recognition are being developed and viewed from the perspective of integrating technologies that can provide highly communicative robots.

Robots are now common "equipment" in medical settings. Active in such settings are machines such as low-fidelity robots that deliver medications to pre-determined areas of the hospital, and surgical robots that assist surgeons for precise surgical procedures [8, 9]. Humanoid robots that can "interact" with humans such as the ASIMO (=Advanced Step in Innovative Mobility, trademarked name) [10] robots produced by Honda can direct patients and visitors to specific areas of the hospital. Multiple human "receptionists" have now been replaced with robotic ones. However, even if robots have begun working in social environments, many issues remain. There are many considerations about development platforms, technical components, safety and responsibility features, and in particular the ethical aspects of care by robots.

Considering whether or not the humanoid nurse robots can be equipped with empathic understanding is deliberated based on findings from a systematic literature review.

2. Examination of prior study

Literature search and review

A systematic review of literature was conducted using SCOPUS as the main search system. A systematic review was conducted using document types such as articles or topic reviews. Key words and number of papers are listed on Tab. 6-1. There are two terms in use, empathetic vs. empathic. According to the website grammarist.com [11], empathic is usually just a variant of empathetic, which means characterized by empathy. Empathic, meanwhile, is commonly found in writing on science and psychology as well as in spiritual and self-help writing. Therefore, this chapter uses the term "empathic".

The terms "empathy", "empathic understanding", "nursing", and "robot", singly or in combination were used as keywords to retrieve related literature published up to the present.

Tab. 6-1: Keywords and number of papers

Keywords	Number of papers
empathy	32,486
empathic and understanding	1,151
nursing and empathy	5,859
nursing and empathic	255
nursing, empathic and understanding	49
robot and emotion	1,969
robot and empathy	157
robot and empathic understanding	11

3. Performance required in nursing robots

3.1. Empathy

There were 32,486 published articles retrieved that used the keyword "empathy" alone. Interestingly, the number of published research was found to be continuously increasing. More than 2000 articles were published in 2012 to 2015 (Fig. 6-1).

Part 2

Most were published in the United States (11,134), followed by those from the United Kingdom (3,325). The focus of research subject areas was from Medicine, which amounted to 30.3% (16,267), followed by Psychology with 17.0% (8,321), Social Sciences with 14.0% (6,587), and Nursing with 9.0% (4,600) (Fig. 6-2).

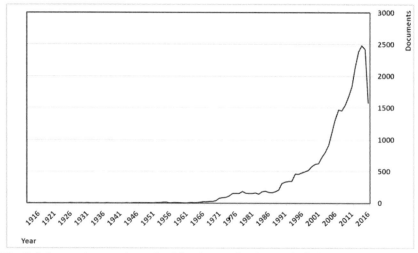

Fig. 6-1: Increasing number of publications using "empathy" alone

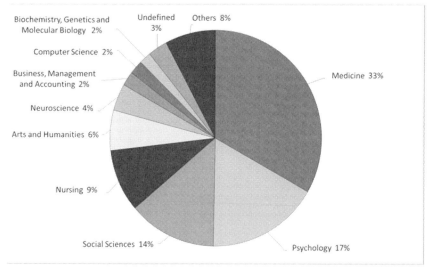

Fig. 6-2: Percentage of publications using "empathy" by research area

The results showed that it was mainly healthcare providers who studied "empathy" instead of those in engineering or psychology.

Recently, studies [12, 13] have defined and described "empathy" as the consequence of neural matching mechanisms comprising a mirror neuron system in the brain. Enabling a person to empathize means he/she can share, or experience the feelings of another person. Moreover, empathy in humans was found to be assisted by other abstract and domain-general high-level cognitive abilities such as executive functions and language, and the ability to differentiate another's mental state from one's own. These expand the range of behaviors that can be driven by empathy. The use of the term "mirroring" is helpful as a loose analogy for the process of "reproducing" the affective experiences of others in our own emotion-related neural systems [14].

3.2. Nursing and empathy

There were 5,859 published articles retrieved using the combined keywords "nursing" and "empathy". There was 1 paper published in 1952, and then, a slow increase in published articles, until the average number reached approximately 200 publications every year after 2004 (Fig. 6-3). Most were published in the United States (1,150), and the United Kingdom (479).

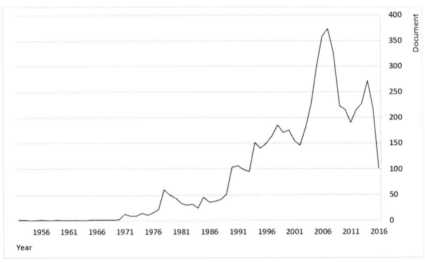

Fig. 6-3: Transitional change of publications using key words "nursing" and "empathy"

"Empathy" [15] is a much debated topic in nursing and medical literature. Because empathy is a complex multi-dimensional concept that has moral cognitive emotive, and behavioral components [16], it involves an ability to understand the patients' situation, perspective, and feelings with their accompanying meanings. Some take the meaning of "empathy" for granted, in that caring and compassion and empathy and sympathy are inclusive, and are often interchangeable terms in nursing [5]. As such, caring, compassion, and empathy are ill-defined [17]. In addition,

Chapter VI

empathy has been variously conceptualized as behavior, a personality dimension, or as an experienced emotion [16].

Therefore, humanoid robot competencies (functions) need to have the ability to empathize in order to contribute to nursing care – to be specific; the robots need the ability to express empathic understanding. As such, further clarification of human-to-human empathic relationships is needed. If the process of empathic understanding could be clarified by a computer program, it is possible to deliberate the abilities of empathic understanding in humanoid robots.

This may be quite feasible these days, for the results of one study showed that communication had four critical themes – one of which was empathy – which results came from McCabe's interviews of patients [18]. Within the nurse-patient relationship empathy was often conceptualized as having a therapeutic value and as such was frequently endorsed as desirable for nursing practice. Some of the latest initiatives aimed at improving the patient's experience include teaching nurses to be more empathic [19], elevating the value of empathy as integral to high quality nursing care, and the value of a trusting relationship between nurse and patients as essential for the growth of patients.

Health service users want the nurse to be skilled technically, and they value his/her being non-judgmental and being patient-centered [20]. Relatedly, real "listening" is not a simple skill, and it is now recognized that communication skills are not innate but need to be taught. Communication skills training aims to teach active listening, empathy, and individual empowerment [21]. It is difficult for nurses to acquire empathetic expressions in nursing. So, human nurses need to train to acquire this skill. In nurse robot-patient relationships, empathic understanding is a critical and essential skill for HNRs.

Furthermore, in Muetzel's model [22] three components of empathy were integrated: namely, partnership, intimacy, and reciprocity. These components coalesce to create a therapeutic relationship. Richardson and others [17] mentioned that Muetzel's model for understanding therapeutic relationships is one framework that can be adopted to help student nurses to appreciate how to build patient

93

Part 2

relationships and encourage them to move towards therapeutic advantage using care, compassion, and empathy. Also, Muetzel's model [17] allows students to consider how nurses would exhibit caring, compassion, and empathy while undertaking common nursing interventions and to use these traits to develop their therapeutic relationship.

In an extensive review of literature on empathy, Morse's model was summarized [16] a conceptual fit for nursing practice components of empathy under four key areas: emotive, moral, cognitive, behavioral. The emotive area is defined as the ability to subjectively experience and share in another's psychological state or intrinsic feelings. The moral is an internal altruistic force that motivates the practice of empathy. The cognitive is the helper's intellectual ability to identify and understand another person's feelings and perspective from an objective stance. The behavioral communicative response to express the understanding of another's perspective conveys the other's understanding of said perspective. From this stance, clinical empathy can be seen as a form of professional interaction competency, rather than a subjective emotional experience or a personality trait that one either has or does not have.

In another study, Barret-Lennard [23] developed a multidimensional model of empathy, referred to as the "empathy cycle", consisting of three phases. Phase 1 is the inner process of empathic listening to another who is personally expressive in some way, and who demonstrates reasoning and understanding; phase 2 is the attempt to convey empathic understanding of the other person's experience; and phase 3 is the client's actual reception or awareness of this communication. Lussier et al. [24] have graphically illustrated this empathic process, based on the research of Barret-Lennard. Such schematization will give important tips for the humanoid robot program.

3.3. Nursing, empathic and understanding

Using a combination of the two critical terms, "nursing" and "empathic", the search revealed 255 related articles. The first research was published in 1966.

94

Afterwards, the year-to-year publication varied considerably. The most that was published were 20 articles in 2012 (Fig. 6-4). Most were published in the United States (56), and the United Kingdom (38).

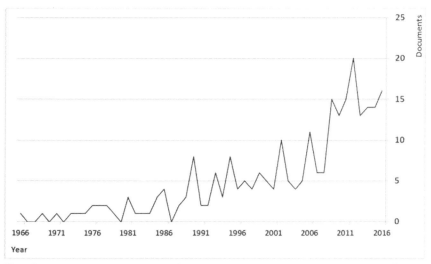

Fig. 6-4: Transitional change of publications using key words "nursing" and "empathic"

Using the three critical terms – "nursing", "empathic", and "understanding" – as keywords revealed 49 articles, with the first being published in 1986. Subsequently, over the years, the numbers of published articles have steadily varied, but 8 articles were published in 2012, with the number varying from 0 to 5 in other years (Fig. 6-5). In descending order of content, 15 were from United Kingdom, 7 from Australia, 4 from the United States.

Part 2

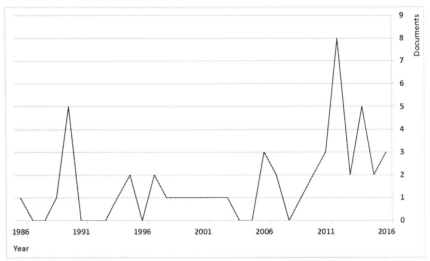

Fig. 6-5: Transitional change of publications using key words "nursing", "empathic", and "understanding"

For example, empathic understanding research for patients with dementia [25] revealed that four key sets of communication skills can support person-centered approaches to dementia care: (1) asking short open questions in the present tense; (2) picking up on emotional cues; (3) giving time and space for the person with dementia to find their words and share responsibility for steering the course of a conversation; and (4) exploring the use of metaphors.

In Japan, robotic conversation research studies on elderly people and patients with dementia showed that conversational robots for dementia prevention [26] and evaluation of robots delaying progression of dementia [27] was possible. Philosopher Metzler [28] describes this as critical for it addresses a topic in nursing philosophy that merits careful attention through dialogue simulation, at the time robots will be introduced to clinical nursing situations.

Cleary, et al. [29] conducted an interview and survey with the results of revealing the importance of communicating accurately and in a timely manner,

Chapter VI

exhibiting empathic understanding with any information of value to patients. In addition, a recent study showed that empathic understanding was critical to the health of patients afflicted by a particular disease [30, 31]. Furthermore, the way of expressing empathic understanding needs to be studied from a sociocultural perspective because of specific sociocultural ways of expression among peoples in different countries [32, 33].

The aforementioned studies support the finding that nurses with expertise in empathic understanding (including comparative cultural knowledge) are able to document the mutual experience with patients well. By analyzing documented data, this will clarify and advance the process of empathic understanding, and help it gain recognition as essential to the human-robot caring practice.

3.4. Robot and the required performance as empathic understanding

There were 1,969 articles retrieved in which "robot" and "emotion" were used as key words. Actually, there were only 496 publications as articles; others were conference papers, editorials, and other forms of academic papers. There were two articles published in 1991. However, there has been an upward trend since 2007 (Fig. 6-6). 77 articles were published in 2013 alone. Most were published in Japan (475), USA (259), and South Korea (164).

Part 2

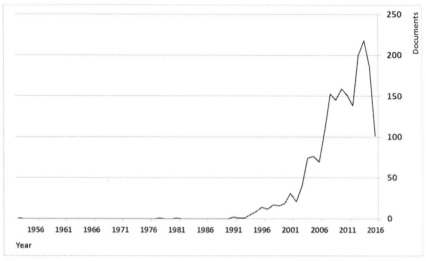

Fig. 6-6: Transitional change of publications using key words "robot" and "emotion"

There were 157 published articles retrieved using the key words "robot" and "empathy". There was 1 paper published in 2000. Depending on the year of publication, the number of published articles ranged from 0 to 9 until 2009. From then on there were over 15 papers published (Fig. 6-7).

Chapter VI

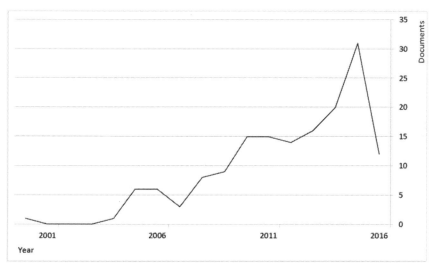

Fig. 6-7: Transitional change of publications using key words "robot" and "empathy"

There was 1 article retrieved in 1986 in which the three keywords "robot", "empathic", and "understanding" were used in combination. A few articles about empathic understanding in robots were found published from 2005.

Research studies focused on empathy for humans to robots [34] or for robots to humans exist, including those studying the educational effect of using robots [35]. It is supposed that robots with empathy or empathic understanding attract attention in the healthcare field. Robots programmed with empathic understanding need to be competent, especially for experimental studies on empathic understanding, as the future unfolds.

It was also found that actions done by other individuals form the stimuli of great importance for primates and humans. If human beings want to survive, humans must understand the actions of others. Furthermore, without action, understanding social organization is impossible [36]. Relative to this brain science approach, potentials are contributing to develop the empathic competence of the human care robot.

Part 2

Furthermore, Nishida, et al. [37] pointed out that sympathy gives a great boost to interaction, and leads to a lively and long-lasting conversation. To build a robot that can create sympathetic relations with human beings, they found that their research was significant in providing robots with the exact dose of intense sympathy. The intensity of robot sympathy varies according to the action of the interactive partner, and affects its own actions.

Robots with empathic understanding need to be able to "understand" and share human emotions so they could be said to possess empathy [38]. To make such a feature possible, roboticists need to endow machines with an empathic module – a software system that can extract emotional cues from human speech and behavior and guides the responses that robots can give accordingly [38].

Expressions of human empathy are combined with facial expressions, conversation, and behavior. The robot extracts emotion from this conversation and behavior, and then, necessarily programs it to respond and act appropriately. Airenti [39] tried to show how developmental psychology may contribute to elucidate artificial empathy.

Research on empathic robots is in its infancy, but scientists are already using signal-processing techniques, machine-learning algorithms, and sentiment analysis tools to build virtual robots that can "understand" human emotion [38]. Jordi Vallverdú and David Casacuberta [40] analyze the ethical challenges of introducing robots into the healthcare field. The challenges become multifactorial when introducing medical machines that are able to understand and mimic human emotions.

The behavior role, function, and electronic circuitry of robots are determined according to an algorithmic "tree structure system" which can be applied to various fields. If a nursing thesaurus can have a "tree structure system" and apply heuristics, there are some possibilities that the expression of empathic understanding in reactive engagements between humans and robots will be realized sooner than later.

100

4. Conclusion

It was clarified that "empathy" in nursing is used as synonym for caring, compassion, and sympathy. In addition, the concept of empathic understanding was drawn from non-nursing (mostly psychology) fields, so that empathy as a nursing practice concept needs to be defined in nursing and its practice. Empathic understanding will become the robot's special feature.

As an active proponent in the front lines of android technologies Ishiguro describes, "I think that it is being a human to believe that there is a mind in each other" [41]. It is thought in engineering that robot research which represents the human empathic understanding is just beginning. In the future, there is a great need to invigorate interdisciplinary collaborative research so it could meet the technological competency and healthcare demands of human caring (Fig. 6-8).

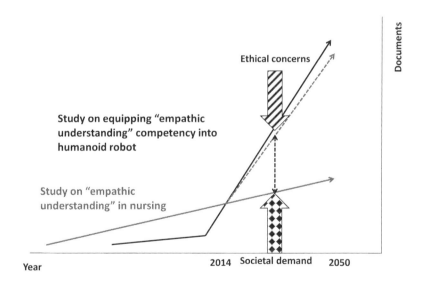

Fig. 6-8: Study on equipping empathic understanding competency into humanoid robot and its future prospects (© Kyoko Osaka)

Part 2

In empathic understanding for robots, assisting healthcare, or in particular, nursing, there are possibilities that a patient's emotion can be supposed from the clear recognition of words he articulates in conversation. Research in natural language processing can be challenged to create demonstrable exercises of prosodic information to assess voice intonation, facial expressions, and other human bodily features that have to do with the particular language used in conversation. A trusting relationship between patient, nurses, robots, and other medical staff is critically important to appreciate empathic communication with the human patient, and to successfully communicate and influence human-robot relationships.

References

[1]   American Association of Critical Care Nurses.
      http://www.aacn.org/wd/hwe/content/aboutassessment.pcms?menu=hwe
      (Accessed 4 January 2016)

[2]   Thornby D: Beginning the Journey to Skilled Communication. AACN Advanced
      critical care, Vol. 17, No. 3, pp. 226-271, 2006.

[3]   Edward Bradford Titchener: Lecture on the Experimental Psychology of
      Thought-Processes. Macmillan, 1909.

[4]   Karsten Stueber: Rediscovering Empathy: Agency, Folk Psychology, and the
      Human Sciences. MIT Press, 2010.

[5]   Dietze E, Orb A: Compassionate care: a moral dimension in nursing. Nursing
      Inquiry, Vol. 7, No. 3, pp. 166-174, 2000.

[6]   Basch MF: Empathic understanding: A review of the concept and some theoretical
      considerations. Journal of the American Psychoanalytic Association, Vol. 31, No. 1,
      pp. 101-126, 1983.

[7]   Rogers C: Reflection of feelings. Person-Centered Review, Vol. 1, pp. 375-377,
      1986.

[8]   Kenngott HG, Wagner M, Nickel F, et al.: Computer-assisted abdominal surgery:
      new technologies. Langenbeck's Archives of Surgery, Vol. 400, No. 3, pp. 273-281,
      2015. DOI: 10.1007/s00423-015-1289-8

Chapter VI

[9] Fisher RA, Dasgupta P, et al.: An over-view of robot assisted surgery curricula and the status of their validation. International Journal of Surgery, Vol. 13, pp. 115-123, 2015. DOI: 10.1016/j.ijsu.2014.11.033

[10] NSTV, Honda's ASIMO robot turns 10. http://www.ndtv.com/photos/news/hondas-asimo-robot-turns-10-8511#photo-104091 (Accessed 20 January 2016)

[11] Grammarist, Empathetic vs. empathic. http://grammarist.com/usage/empathetic-empathic/ (Accessed 29 November 2016)

[12] Decety J, Jackson PL: A social-neuroscience perspective on empathy. Current Directions in Psychological Science, Vol. 15, pp. 54-58, 2006.

[13] Gallese V: The roots of empathy: The Shared Manifold Hypothesis and the Neural Basis of Intersubjectivity. Psychopathology, Vol. 36, pp. 171-180, 2003.

[14] Lamma C, Majdandzic J: The role of shared neural activations, mirror neurons, and morality in empathy- A critical comment. Neuroscience Research, Vol. 90, pp. 15-24, 2015. DOI: 10.1016/j.neures.2014.10.008.

[15] Dinkins CS: Ethics: Beyond patient care: Practicing empathy in the workplace. The Online Journal of Issues in nursing, Vol. 16, No. 2, 2011. http://www.nursingworld.org/MainMenuCategories/ANAMarketplace/ANAPeriodicals/OJIN/Columns/Ethics/Empathy-in-the-Workplace.html (Accessed 22 January 2016)

[16] Mercer SW, Reynolds WJ: Empathy and quality of care. The British Journal of General Practice, Vol. 52, Supp l, pp. 9-12, 2002.

[17] Richardson C, Percy M, Hughes J: Nursing therapeutic: Teaching student nurses care compassion and empathy. Nursing Education Today, Vol.35, No.5, pp. 1-5, 2015. DOI: 10.1016/j.nedt.2015.01.016

[18] McCabe C: Nurse-patient communication: an exploration of patients' experiences. Journal of Clinical Nursing, Vol. 13, No. 1, pp.41-49, 2004. DOI: 10.1111/j.1365-2702.2004.00817.x

103

Part 2

[19] Yu J, Kirk M: Measurement of empathy in nursing research: systematic review. Journal of Advanced Nursing, Vol. 64, No. 5, pp. 440-454, 2008. DOI: 10.1111/j.1365-2648.2008.04831.x

[20] Griffithsm J, Speed S, Horne M, Keeley P: 'A caring professional attitude': What service users and carers seek in graduate nurses and the challenge for educators. Nurse Education Today, Vol. 32, No. 2, pp. 121-127, 2012. DOI: 10.1016/j.nedt.2011.06.005

[21] Maguire P, Pitceathly C: Key communication skills and how to acquire them. British Medical Journal, Vol. 325, No. 7366, pp. 697-700, 2002.

[22] Muetzel PA: Therapeutic nursing. In Primary Nursing, Nursing in the Burford and Oxford Nursing Development Units, (Pearson, A. ed.), Chapman & Hall, pp.89-116, 1988.

[23] Barrett-Lennard GT: The empathy cycle: Refinement of a nuclear concept. Journal of Counseling Psychology, Vol. 28, No. 2, pp. 91-100, 1981.

[24] Lussier MT, Richard C: Reflecting back: Empathic process. Canadian Family Physician, Vol. 53, No. 5, pp. 827-828, 2007.

[25] Mcevoy P, Plant R: Dementia care: Using empathic curiosity to establish the common ground that is necessary for meaningful communication. Journal of Psychiatric and Mental Health Nursing, Vol. 21, No. 6, pp. 477-482, 2014. DOI: 10.1111/jpm.12148

[26] Oida Y, Kanoh M: Practice of the care prevention that utilized a robot. Japan society of nursing, welfare and health promotion, Vol. 1, No. 2, pp. 95-99, 2014.

[27] Izutsu Y, Sumiyoshi R, Kawanaka H, Yamamoto K, Suzuki K, Takase H, Tsuruoka S: A proposal of dementia evaluation method using interaction with communication robots in welfare facilities. Japan association for medical informatics, Vol. 32, No. 2, pp. 83-93, 2012. DOI: http://doi.org/10.14948/jami.32.83

[28] Metzler TA, Barnes SJ: Three dialogues concerning robots in elder care. Nursing Philosophy, Vol. 15, No. 1, pp. 4-13, 2014. DOI: 10.1111/nup.12027

Chapter VI

[29] Cleary M, Hunt GE, Escott P, Walter G: Receiving Difficult News. Views of patients in an inpatient setting. Journal of Psychosocial Nursing and Mental Health Services, Vol. 48 No. 6, pp. 40-48, 2010.

[30] Pollard C, Fitzgerald M, Ford K: Delirium: The lived experience of older people who are delirious post-orthopaedic surgery. International Journal of Mental Health Nursing, Vol. 24, No. 3, pp. 213-221, 2015. DOI: 10.1111/inm.12132

[31] Probst S, Arber A, Faithfull S: Malignant fungating wounds – The meaning of living in an unbounded body. European Journal of Oncology Nursing, Vol. 17, No. 1, pp. 38-45, 2013. DOI: 10.1016/j.ejon.2012.02.001

[32] Hawamdeh S, Hawamdeh S: Exploring empathy: A perspective of Arab nurses. World Applied Sciences Journal, Vol. 17, No. 6, pp. 786-791, 2012.

[33] Rchaidia L, Dierckx de Casterlé B, Verbeke G, Gastmans C: Oncology patients' perceptions of the good nurse: An explorative study on the psychometric properties of the Flemish adaptation of the Care-Q instrument. Journal of Clinical Nursing, Vol. 21, No. 9-10, pp. 1387-1400, 2012. DOI: 10.1111/j.1365-2702.2011.03861.x

[34] Suzuki Y, Galli L, Ikeda A, et al.: Measuring empathy for human and robot hand pain using electroencephalography. Scientific report, Vol. 5, 15924, 2015. http://www.nature.com/articles/srep15924, 2016.1.22 access

[35] Han J, Jo M, Hyun E, So H: Examining young children's perception toward augmented reality-influenced dramatic play. Educational Technology Research and Development, Vol. 63, No. 3, pp. 455-474, 2015. DOI: 10.1007/s11423-015-9374-9

[36] Rizzolatti G, Craighero L: The Mirror Neuron System. Annual Review of Neuroscience, Vol. 27, pp. 169-192, 2004.
DOI: 10.1146/annurev.neuro.27.070203.144230

[37] Nishida R, Nagai T, et al.: Interaction with a Sympathetic Robot. Human-Agent International Symposium 2013, Gifu, pp. 117-119, 2013. (In Japanese)

[38] Fung P: Robot with heart. How to build an empathetic robot. Scientific American, Vol. 313, pp. 61-63, 2015. DOI:10.1038/scientificamerican1115-60

105

Part 2

[39] Airenti G: The Cognitive Bases of Anthropomorphism: From Relatedness to Empathy. International journal of social robotics, Vol. 7, No. 1, pp. 117-127, 2015. DOI: 10.1007/s12369-014-0263-x

[40] Vallverdú J, Casacuberta D: Ethical and Technical Aspects of Emotions to Create Empathy in Medical Machines. Machine Medical Ethics, Vol. 74, pp. 341-362, 2014. DOI: 10.1007/978-3-319-08108-3_20

[41] Ishiguro H: What is robot — mirror of the mind —. Kodansha's new library of knowledge, Kodansha Ltd. 2009. (In Japanese)

Abstract

This chapter considers the implications of Natural Language Processing (NLP) in human interactions, and explains contemporary issues and conditions influencing the development and required level of appreciating NLP for a humanoid nurse robot.

Key Words: Empathic understanding, Nnursing, Nurse-robot, Communication, Caring

Chapter VII

The Current State of Performance and Development of Natural Language Processing Required for Humanoid Caring Robots

By Kazuyuki Matsumoto

Part 2

1. Introduction

In recent years, humanoid robots that can handle natural language have been put into practical use (e.g., Pepper [1], NAO [2], PALRO [3]). These robots are capable of making conversation with people by using human languages. In nursing care, communication with patients is an important factor and one of its most important issues is the application of communication techniques to nursing robots.

This chapter summarizes the artificial intelligence-based dialogue system that is recently gathering attention as a Natural Language Processing (NLP) technique applicable to a care robot. Also, this chapter refers to the robust language understanding methods that deal with the unknown expressions that appear in dialogue, and points out several noticeable issues when implementing these methods in care robots.

2. Current stage of natural language processing for care robot – dialogue system based on artificial intelligence techniques

In recent natural language processing situations dealing with robots, the most remarkable field is the dialogue processing system based on artificial intelligence techniques. The core of recent artificial intelligence techniques is machine learning methods such as the deep learning technique. In this technique, a large amount of data (i.e., "big data") is used, which data used to be considered impossible to process due to hardware constraints. However, this is no longer true because sufficient hardware resources are now relatively easy to prepare and secure.

This section introduces the existing studies or services that realize dialogue processing by analyzing natural language based on a large amount of data, using these machine learning methods. Following are some examples:

108

Chapter VII

・ Apple "Siri" [4]

Speech Interpretation and Recognition Interface (Siri) is an artificial intelligence software with a speech assistance functionality developed for iOS or macOS Sierra. The system responds to the questions inputted by the user's voice using NLP. This has been implemented in the iPhone, one of Apple's major products, acquiring a high degree of public recognition.

・ Microsoft "Rinna" [5]

The system is a chatbot running on the LINE social networking service. The system is characterized by a chatbot called Rinna, whose personality is programmed as a high school girl. A user can communicate with Rinna through chat. The system uses big data on "Bing" (a search engine developed by Microsoft) and social networking sites as training data. It is based on a dialogue engine constructed using a machine learning platform called "Azure Machine Learning".

・ NTT Docomo chat API [6]

The chat dialogue API provided by NTT Docomo Developer Support can recognize natural dialogue from a user's spoken text, using NLP. Compared to the previous voice assistance techniques dealing with task-based dialogue, this API was created for non-task-based dialogue.

・ Deep LSTM chatbot (Seq2Seq) [7]

Recently, Deep Learning has received a lot of attention as a technique as well as for its artificial intelligence. Deep Learning was developed from a neural network, and the technique finally bloomed in the current age of big data and its accompanying advancement in rapid processing techniques such as GPGPU. Seq2Seq is an algorithm that can convert a character string into another character string by using a kind of recurrent neural network called Long Short-Term Memory (LSTM) [8]. This algorithm is expected to be applied to machine translation. In

109

Part 2

addition, by considering dialogue as the translation process of interpreting an utterance and generating its response, the algorithm also focuses on dialogue.

Recent studies on dialogue systems pursue the "humanity" that is required to process dialogue in nursing care. At the same time, the problems of artificial intelligence (AI) are gathering attention; for example, dialogue systems using AI technology could speak something unethical (e.g. revealing private patient information to others), which we call a "runaway of AI". There is a high risk involved in using the knowledge obtained by machine learning based on big data, and it is a risk too huge for us to grasp without manual checking.

Therefore, it was considered a need to check the knowledge used for nursing care either manually or by automatically filtering the nursing care knowledge based on ethical norms. The nursing care robots currently used for clinical trials can handle only simple dialogue. However, it is expected that such a time will come, probably in the near future, that patients can enjoy conversation with nursing care robots as if they were humans.

The author thinks that advanced intelligent robots possessing artificial intelligence techniques have personalities. If he put a nursing care robot to work without preparing a system to train that robot, which system is based on high ethical standards, he will surely have difficulties in handling that new member of the labor force.

3. Natural language understanding: Robust to unknown expressions

Recently, the opportunities to post comments have been increasing on microblogs such as weblogs or Twitter. Many of these comments (i.e., short text) include the writers' feelings at that time or opinions toward something. However, it would be difficult to understand the meanings of such short texts, from such a variety of users, without using a dictionary including all the expressions used on microblogs.

Chapter VII

On the other hand, nursing care robots must have an ability to estimate the emotions of their patients from information such as words, gestures or facial expressions. This section describes the outline of an emotion corpus being constructed by the author's research group on how to estimate the emotional state of the patients via that corpus, and it also explains a method to expand the emotion corpus. In addition, this section introduces our proposed techniques to estimate emotional states from utterances with unknown expressions not registered in the dictionary, with corresponding examples.

The research groups by Ren et al. are engaged in constructing the emotion corpora.

Ren-CECps [9, 10] is a large-scale text corpus consisting of Chinese weblog articles. The corpus has manual annotations of eight kinds of emotions and their strength is based on article, paragraph, and word. Ren and Matsumoto [11] also constructed a slang emotion corpus. This corpus collected the sentences including youth slang and annotated emotion tags on the sentences. The validity of both corpora was evaluated through the emotion classification experiments using the machine learning method.

Matsumoto, et al. [12] proposed a method to quantize the words into their concepts as a framework that can deal with the sentences, including unknown words. Some studies have already proposed the methods to convert words into their distributed expressions, and sentiment analysis was one of their applications. In this research, the existing classification method that was based on machine learning and that used the "Bag of Words" as a feature could increase its accuracy by refining the number of concepts and by using instead a "Bag of Concepts". The proposed method considered two kinds of weighting of the feature. One used concept frequency as weight. The other weighted the feature according to the degree to which a word belonged to each concept.

Fig. 7-1 shows the result of emotion estimation based on the k-nearest neighbor method and the concept quantization. The concept quantization method based on the corpus collected by emotional expression as a key was more effective

111

Part 2

than the method based on the corpus collected by unknown expression as a key. Limiting the target to the kinds of emotions recognizable by a nursing care robot brought about the consideration that accurate classification is expected more.

The corpus-based method has a problem caused by annotation variance. If the tag annotation standard is changed a little, a completely different corpus would be made; as a result, the estimation result would differ. To solve this problem, we should simplify the annotation work and take a measure to limit the corpus, for example, only to the corpus based on the actual dialogue data recorded in a nursing facility.

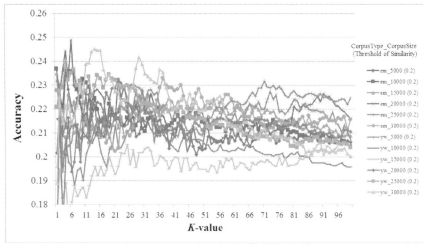

Fig. 7-1: Comparison of emotion estimation accuracies by k-nearest neighbor method based on concept quantization

4. Problems of implementation in a nursing care robot

This section describes the problems to be solved to implement NLP in a nursing care robot.

112

Chapter VII

4.1. Improper words

A technique is required that can automatically recognize rude or improper words spoken to the user (the person who receives care) and then ban them.

4.2. Unnatural words

As one of the voice synthesis techniques, a technique to realize fluent phonation has been developed along with the advancement of recent machine learning methods. However, people sometimes use unnatural and ungrammatical language. Therefore, by reproducing even such natural errors, the system can make users feel as if they were talking with a real person.

4.3. Training function

When a nursing robot is designed to construct linguistic knowledge for each user independently, the robot would contain several different personalities, each with its own unique linguistic knowledge. It would be difficult for the administrator (supervisor) to train each personality in a nursing robot individually. Therefore, a mechanism would be required that can coordinate the basic personality of the nursing robot and the user-adaptive personalities.

5. Conclusion

With the development of dialogue processing systems, intelligent dialogue processing by robots will be improved continually. It is easy to imagine that the problems of dialogue processing systems could then be overcome in nursing robots. The NLP techniques uniquely developed for a nursing robot might be applied to other systems in the future.

The discussion on NLP for nursing robots has only just begun. It is difficult for engineering researchers to imagine precisely what problems might occur in actual nursing situations. It is necessary to set up a multidisciplinary research team to realize and develop nursing robots with advanced linguistic functions.

113

Part 2

References

[1] Softbank: Pepper. http://www.softbank.jp/robot/consumer/products/ (in Japanese)

[2] ALDEBARAN NAO: An Introduction to Robotics with NAO. http://www.hamiltoncentral.org/cms/lib011/NY01947832/Centricity/Domain/81/AnIntroductionToRoboticsWithNao_TextBook_2012_US.pdf

[3] FUJISOFT: Palro Academic Series. https://palro.jp/pdf/acade.pdf

[4] APPLE: Siri. http://www.apple.com/jp/ios/siri/ (in Japanese)

[5] Microsoft: Rinna. http://rinna.jp/ (in Japanese)

[6] NTT Docomo: chat API. https://dev.smt.docomo.ne.jp/?p=docs.api.page&api_name=dialogue&p_name=api_reference (in Japanese)

[7] Ilya S, Oriol V, Quoc VL: Sequence to Sequence Learning with Neural Networks. Advances in Neural Information Processing Systems 27. Curran Associates, Inc., pp.3104-3112, 2014.

[8] Hochreiter S, Schmidhuber I: Long short-term memory. Neural Computation, 1997.

[9] Li J, Ren F: Creating a Chinese emotion lexicon based on corpus Ren-CECps. Proceedings of 2011 IEEE International Conference on Cloud Computing and Intelligence Systems (CCIS), pp. 15-17, 2011.

[10] Quan C, Ren F: Recognizing sentence emotions based on polynomial kernel method using Ren-CECps. Proceedings of International Conference on Natural Language Processing and Knowledge Engineering. NLP-KE 2009, pp. 24-27, 2009.

[11] Ren F, Matsumoto K: Semi-Automatic Creation of Youth Slang Corpus and Its Application to Affective Computing. IEEE Transactions on Affective Computing, Vol.7, Issue 2, pp. 176-189, 2016.

[12] Matsumoto K, Yoshida M, Xiao O, Luo X, Kita K: Emotion recognition for sentences with unknown expressions based on semantic similarity by using Bag of Concepts. In Proceedings of the 12th International Conference on Fuzzy Systems and Knowledge Discovery (FSKD2015), pp. 15-17, 2015.

Abstract

This chapter describes and explains the kinds of emotion recognition technologies (including expression recognition, speech recognition, and natural language processing) demanded by human beings in order to accept a humanoid nurse robot.

Key Words: Healthcare, Robotics, Population reduction, Aging society

Chapter VIII

Natural Language Processing Capabilities Required for Humanoid Nursing Robots

By Fuji Ren, Kazuyuki Matsumoto

Part 2

1. Introduction

When humans communicate with each other, they try to convey intention or emotion by using language, gesture, facial expression, and voice [1-8]. Among these, it is the reliance of human emotion on psychological elements that can give engineering researchers trouble understanding exactly what kinds of problems they may encounter in their communication. On the other hand, uses for practical communication robots are universally recognized in ordinary society. The techniques that can be applied to intelligent dialogue represent a major advance in artificial intelligence, natural language processing, speech recognition technique, and computer vision.

Generally, it is hoped that communication robots can express/recognize emotion in the same way as humans. However, in nursing care, caretakers must include emotional labor. They must recognize their patients' emotional states through small/little changes, while containing their own emotions. If a patient's mental state is unbalanced, the patient – in the worst case – could potentially commit suicide. Therefore, we must consider early detection of depressive tendencies, which can be a factor in suicidal tendencies. Working mainly from web blog articles, this chapter introduces the proposed framework for emotion recognition, and depression tendency detection in robots.

2. Recognition of human emotions

In traditional behavioral psychology, researchers deal with the recognition of human emotions; however, engineering methods have not yet been established. Nevertheless, artificial intelligence researchers have already been working on an information processing method based on the human psyche and human culture, although the researchers have yet to make a machine that can recognize and represent human emotions. These previous studies have not focused on the depth of the human mind and thus have not yet achieved recognition of human emotions.

Chapter VIII

Here, we briefly describe the Mental State Transition Network (MSTN) as the emotion recognition framework. External input such as linguistic information and facial expressions are not enough to model human emotional states. It is necessary to combine these with more physically recognizable reactions. It is hypothesized that human emotions are placed in transit between several discrete states, which are defined as "mental states". Analysis of a huge amount of data and human individual characteristics information allows us to build the following network modules representing mental state transitions, as shown in Fig. 8-1. In Fig. 8-1, 0 means Serene, 1 means Happy, 2 means Sad, 3 means Angry, 4 means Disgust, 5 means Fear and 6 means Surprise.

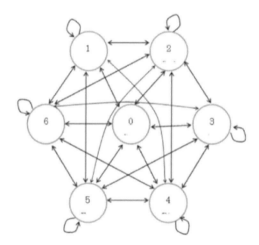

Fig. 8-1: Concept of Mental State Transition Network (MSTN)

3. Depression-tendency detection by emotion recognition

The estimation of a patient's emotional state from various situations is useful to assess the mental health of the patient. This section introduces the method to detect depressive signs in patients as an approach to enriching the human mind in

Part 2

the "Enriching Mental Engineering" method proposed by the authors [9, 10]. Complaints of depression and anxiety are very common among adult patients seeking treatment in primary care settings. Appropriate therapy or medicine is required because each patient represents a different situation. It is thought that depression is difficult to recover from fully, because there are no clear symptoms associated with the condition. It is vital that persons close to those at risk watch for indications, and encourage sufferers to get counseling or early therapy before the disorder progresses.

The proposed method detects weblog writers who have depressive tendencies based on the emotional fluctuation that can be recognized from their articles. First, we classified the weblog users into depressive/non-depressive, and counted the number of articles posted by each user. Next, the weblog articles were annotated manually with emotion tags.

In this study, we aggregated these emotion tags at regular intervals, converted the positive/negative fluctuation features to the vectors, and constructed the classifier to discriminate between depression and non-depression. A part of the experiment is shown in Fig. 8-2. This study achieved some accuracy of detection of depression and non-depression; these results were obtained in the dataset. Actually, because it is quite unlikely that the number of the users who have depressive tendencies or are non-depressive is half-and-half, it is critically required to validate the realistic distributed conditions.

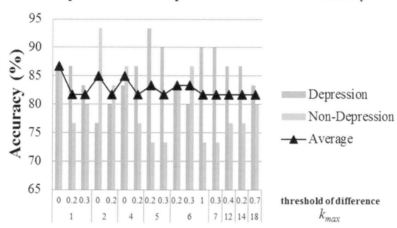

Fig. 8-2: The judgment result based on estimated emotional fluctuation pattern vector

4. Prototype of humanoid robot

We constructed the humanoid emotional robot as the prototype of a nursing robot. The robot shown in Fig. 8-3 can understand human language and recognize/express emotions. This is the existing robot "Robovie R-2" that was programmed with an emotion recognition engine, and which can recognize linguistic/voice emotion and facial expression. Then, the robot decides and expresses a self-emotion state based on the MSTN. The robot shown in Fig. 8-4 is an Actroid made in the image of a person.

We try to recognize and extract emotional information from linguistic information, facial expression, and voice. In future work, we would like to conduct various preliminary experiments to use for clinical investigation in an actual care environment.

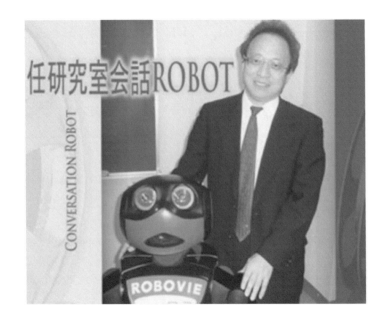

Fig. 8-3: Humanoid robot implemented with emotion recognition engine and emotion expression mechanism

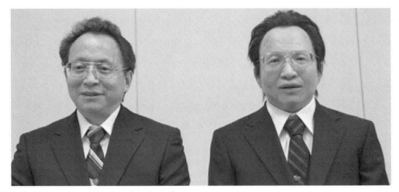

Fig. 8-4: Humanoid robot "Actroid"

Chapter VIII

5. Conclusion

In this chapter – taking into consideration an important method in nursing care to recognize human emotion – the authors' research group introduced a part of their proposed emotion recognition engine and a detection method for use with subjects displaying depressive tendencies. Although human emotion recognition is important for providing care, further study is required from new perspectives that are different from existing studies of communication robots. It is also necessary to discuss how to control the emotion representation by a robot from the aspect of emotional labor in the future.

Acknowledgments

This research was partially supported by JSPS KAKENHI Grant Numbers 15H01712.

References

[1] Ren F: Affective Information Processing and Recognizing Human Emotion. Electronic Notes in Theoretical Computer Science, Vol. 225, No. 2009, pp. 39-50, 2009.

[2] Matsumoto K, Yoshida M, Tsuchiya S, Kita K, Ren F: Slang Analysis Based on Variant Information Extraction Focusing on the Time Series Topics. International Journal of Advanced Intelligence (IJAI), Vol. 8, No. 1, pp. 84-98, 2016.

[3] Ren F, Wu Y: Predicting User-topic Opinions in Twitter with Social and Topical Context. IEEE Transactions on Affective Computing, (10.1109/T-AFFC.2013.22), Vol. 4, No. 4, pp. 412-424, 2013.

[4] Quan C, Ren F: Weighted high-order hidden Markov models for compound emotions recognition in text. Information Sciences, Vol. 329, pp. 581-596, 2015. DOI: 10.1016/j.ins.2015.09.050

Part 2

[5] Ren F, Huang Z: Facial expression recognition based on AAM-SIFT and adaptive regional weighting. IEEJ Transactions on Electrical and Electronic Engineering, 2015. DOI: 10.1002/tee.22151

[6] Quan C, Ren F: Textual Emotion Recognition for Enhancing Enterprise Computing. Enterprise Information Systems, August, 2014.
DOI: 10. 1080/17517575.2014.948935

[7] Ren F, Kan X: Employing Hierarchical Bayesian Networks in Simple and Complex Emotion Topic Analysis, Computer Speech and Language, Vol. 27, pp. 943-968, 2013. DOI: 10.1016/j.csl.2012.07.012

[8] Ren F, Matsumoto K: Semi-automatic Creation of Youth Slang Corpus and Its Application to Affective Computing. IEEE Transactions on Affective Computing, 2015. DOI: 10.1109/TAFFC.2015.2457915

[9] Ren F, Quan C, Matsumoto K: ENRICHING MENTAL ENGINEERING. International Journal of Innovative Computing, Information and Control, Vol. 9, No. 8, pp. 3271-3286, 2013.

[10] Ren F, Kang X, Quan C: Examining Accumulated Emotional Traits in Suicide Blogs with an Emotion Topic Model. IEEE Journal of Biomedical and Health Informatics, 2015. DOI:10.1109/JBHI.2015.2459683

122

Abstract

This chapter describes the underpinnings of the caring nature and treatment in transactive relationships among psychiatrist or family physician, patient, family, and the Care Robot Trio "SHIN-GI-TAI"; narrative knowing, and the use of situated virtual stories of professional practice. These explain caring and treatment activities used by the healthcare robots in Tanioka's Transactive Relationship Theory of Nursing (TRETON).

Key Words: Care Robot Trio "SHIN-GI-TAI", Artificial intelligence, Elderly mental healthcare, Psychiatrists, Transactive relationships

Chapter IX

The Care Robot Trio "SHIN-GI-TAI" in 2050:

Transactive Relations among Psychiatrist, Patient, and

Family

**By Yueren Zhao, Tetsuya Tanioka, Rozzano C. Locsin,
Kyoko Osaka, Yuko Yasuhara**

Part 2

1. Introduction

In 2035, the highly advanced information society will emerge and will continue to progress like "greedy growing creatures". This advancement is due mainly to a dramatic advancement in information technology (IT) [1]. At the same time, the aging society of countries such as Japan continues to advance to the category of a "super-aged society" which requires multidisciplinary collaboration and training for the promotion of better healthcare [2]. How will this healthcare be practiced in situations concerning the advanced older patient and his family? How will psychiatrists and nurses practice and engage in these patients' healthcare scenarios using the Care Robot Trio "SHIN-GI-TAI"? In the new era of greedy capitalism – where desires rule society – terms such as efficiency priority, profit priority, and permanent ownership monopoly at the highly advanced information society in the super-aged society is necessary in order to blend Western wisdom and Oriental ethics for the realization of personal dignity-based mental healthcare.

This chapter describes the underpinnings of the caring nature and treatment in transactive relationships among psychiatrist or family physician, patient, family, and the Care Robot Trio "SHIN-GI-TAI"; narrative knowing, and the use of situated virtual stories [3] of professional practice. These explain caring and treatment activities used by the healthcare robots in the Transactive Relationship Theory of Nursing (TRETON) (Tanioka, 2017) [4].

It is critically important that the contributing factors that impact the delivery and functionality of the practice are clearly described and appreciated. These factors as concepts of care are influenced by Theraveda Buddhist teachings.

The Theravada Buddhist teachings: The challenge for self-awareness

Persons are responsive individuals whose characteristics embody their humanness. The teachings of Buddha pertain to these characteristics and allow healthcare workers to appreciate a person in relation to others [5]. For healthcare providers, the practice of caring and the practice of purifying one's spirit of evil

124

Chapter IX

thought (cleansing the mind) here is almost the same practice. This will not change in either 2017 or 2050.

The Care Robot Trio "SHIN-GI-TAI" here shows the importance of a healthcare provider doing actions of self-understanding (or self-awareness) as a human being.

The three characteristics of Impermanence (Anicca), Suffering (Dukkha), and Egolessness (Anatta) make it possible for human behaviors to cause a shift once healthcare workers are able to reflect on these behaviors. Attempting to combine the philosophical viewpoint of Theravada Buddhism with the idea of patient-centered caring, one can identify three essential characteristics as the cause of Suffering (Dukkha) from the teachings of the Buddha and the possibilities of monitoring the Three Roots [6] of being unskilled, i.e. "TON, greed (lobha)", "JIN, rejecting and anger (dosa)", and "CHI, ignoring and laziness (moha)". However, there are also three coping behaviors for each of these roots, i.e. Sharing, Loving-Kindness, and Mindfulness. These coping behaviors are described, explained, and proposed as critical ways to knowing persons, as well as addressing healthcare problems.

2. Care Robot Trio "SHIN-GI-TAI"

This Care Robot Trio is a blueprint for the upcoming prediction that the intelligent machines possessing artificial intelligence (AI) will be able to interact with humans in 2050. This projects the future idea of human caring from the viewpoint of using high-tech care with the Care Robots among transactive relations.

What is the SHIN-GI-TAI:

The SHIN-GI-TAI is an AI/Robot Care System. It is not a stand-alone supercomputer system, rather it is a single unit of AI/Robots, a "virtual professional team" operated by a physician at the scene. However, SHIN-GI-TAI will be performing as a networked AI/Robot unit "plugged into 7 billion human minds, plus quintillions of online transistors, plus hundreds of exabytes of real-life data, plus the

125

Part 2

self-correcting feedback loops of the entire civilization" [7]. To appreciate the workings of the SHIN-GI-TAI, the following descriptions are presented.

"SHIN" has many kinds of physical sensors for monitoring a psychiatrist's physical and mental conditions. It is simultaneously connected to GI and TAI using advanced wireless technologies. A pair of virtual reality (VR) glasses inscribed with the term SHIN and/or a VR contact lens also inscribed with SHIN are available. The neural network AI instantly analyzes the physical and mental information monitored by SHIN, and will be fed back on-site tutorials through the companion AI/robot "GI".

"GI" (Amedeo) is a VR avatar-type AI/Robot. It also has many kinds of physical sensors for monitoring patients' physical and mental statuses. It is simultaneously connected to a Neural Network Center using advanced wireless technologies. GI is also a downloadable VR avatar, so operators may easily get clones anywhere and anytime, particularly when individual authentications are done correctly through the Neural Network environment.

"TAI" is a term of aggregation of AI/Robots controlled by advanced "internet of things (IoT)" technologies. TAIs usually belong to the patients or to their communities, but the psychiatrist, or the operators of the SHIN-GI-TAI, are allowed to connect, control, and use TAIs on-site through the wirelessly connected VR avatar "GI". TAI has so many formations such as full-automatic vehicle-type AI/robots that are called "cars" today, fully-automatic cooking AI/robots called "microwaves" or "fridges", or wearable universal multi-posture supporting AI/robots called "wheelchairs".

This virtual caring situation is a blueprint for the prediction that the "encounter between people" included in this situation will revolve around the elements of caring and ethical issues in 2050. The theory of caring used to center only on the Western way of thinking, but in this chapter the authors aim to introduce Oriental Buddhist thinking into new conceptualizations of caring theory. This chapter projects human caring from the viewpoint of using the high-tech care of the Care Robots and their transactive relations with healthcare participants. In the future

126

Chapter IX

it is speculated that the environments of the virtual and actual realities can exist together. Also, the benefits and risks of scientific and technological progress that can occur in the surroundings of the future patient (region, environment, people, etc.) are considered.

3. The importance of healthcare practices based on caring partnership among persons and healthcare robots

The older population will have increased dramatically by 2035, and by that time, these super-aged persons will require increased mental healthcare settings, which could result in serious healthcare staffing shortages [8]. With the elimination and consolidation of mental health institutions and facilities in the community steadily progressing through medical welfare-related budgets, another factor that could drastically increase the population of older persons is the progress in gene therapy and nanotechnology [9]. By the authors' projection, there are possibilities that many people facing the new challenging prospect of increased "longevity" will be seeking mental healthcare.

Even if the development of a highly advanced information society expands appropriate knowledge about mental disorders, it is unlikely that the social stigma for people with mental disorders and mental healthcare will be easily alleviated or eliminated [10, 11]. Alongside advances in mental healthcare, cooperation among not only other healthcare providers but also among public health nurses, associate persons, educators, etc. is needed where collaboration becomes required [12]. There is Western thought that puts emphasis on absolute values, as seen in Evidence Based Medicine (EBM); however, no single model for organizing the incorporation of EBM is fully satisfactory [13]. Perhaps, in the next millennium, one of the aims of evidence-based healthcare practice will be the purification of human minds by noticing greed, anger, and ignorance deep in the human heart.

The expected effects are better reflections and personal interactions [14]. A caring partnership among person-person and person-healthcare robot will be needed.

127

Part 2

4. Rationalizing the influence of Buddhist thought in practice

The biggest reason for focusing on the teaching of Buddha comes from the realization of the way the mind works in the case of a medical staff who is "handling" healthcare robots and caring for users of robots. That is, the attempt to "center oneself" and empty the mind, calm the soul, and allow clinical attitudes that encompass humility, selflessness, compassion, and conscience to enter the mind and usher into oneness with the patients' universe in caring situations.

With the Care Robot Trio "SHIN-GI-TAI", the medical staff can perform human healthcare while purifying themselves. The profound changes this purification brings in the attitudes of medical staff may also influence those receiving healthcare to purify themselves as well, and experience the same changes. Centering oneself becomes an effective way to focus on the problem at hand. This influence of Buddhist thought makes it critically important to focus and clear the mind at the beginning of each caring nursing event.

In highly advanced societies, there ought to be an educated and qualified mental healthcare staff to promote further collaboration, not only with other healthcare specialists but also with other stakeholders in the community, including the residents, public health agents, education officials, and others. While caring for super-aged persons, medical personnel must deal with their own aging problem as well. There is no guarantee that securing health services and financial resources that can frequently enforce visits and visiting rights of nursing personnel by a multi-disciplinary team will always be possible.

Nevertheless, major reforms are continually being implemented in Japan's medical and nursing care systems, and the basic pension system of the elderly has maintained the public healthcare insurance system. The more the country faces big challenges – i.e., the lack of medical personnel and suppression of welfare-related budgets – the more extensively we explore new ideas, using up-to-date and advancing technologies, of promoting fair and equitable elderly mental healthcare in the super-aged society. Of course, open-minded clinical ideas with high versatility

128

Chapter IX

that can be handled are required, not only for the elderly but also for all generations.

5. Issues concerning the Care Robot Trio "SHIN-GI-TAI"

Applications of care technologies and how these work in practice, i.e. mimicking the performance of human interactions, specifically intelligent machines possessing AI, are discussed below.

The terms "心 (SHIN: spirit), 技 (GI: technology), and 体 (TAI: body)" are the concepts most important in supporting mental healthcare professionals who will have started seeing patients at the scene by 2035. The Care Robot Trio "SHIN-GI-TAI" is supporting medical personnel with aging problems as a part of fair, equitable, and open-minded medical practice.

In Japanese, "心 (SHIN)" stands for "mind" or "mental activity". Through the following functions, SHIN supports compassionate and ethical medical practice.

5.1. Wearable type AI/Robot: 心 (SHIN)

SHIN is a wearable virtual reality tool that looks like eyeglasses, consisting of two ultra-small high-performance video cameras, a lens with a monitor display screen function, and a microphone and earphone attached to a next-generation communication system without solid batteries. The two ultra-small high-performance video cameras – one inward-facing and the other outward-facing – are mounted on the bridge of the eyeglasses. The outward-facing camera is for taking pictures and recording videos of clinical sites while the inward-facing camera is for monitoring various physiological responses, including the doctor's pupil diameter, the skin around the eyes, the arrector pili muscle, and capillary blood vessels.

The SHIN has sensors embedded in the eyeglasses, its frame, and its nose pad that monitor physiological responses such as the owner's skin temperature, the psychiatrists' measures of "TON 貪 (greed)", "JIN 瞋 (rejecting and anger)", and

129

Part 2

"Chi 痴 (ignoring and laziness)", in conjunction with the inward-facing camera (Fig.9-1).

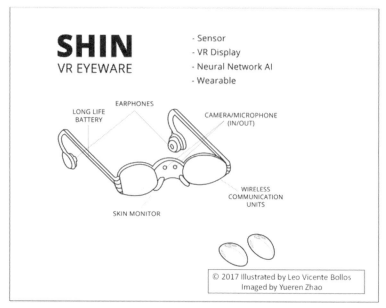

Fig. 9-1: Wearable type AI/Robot: 心 (SHIN)

The SHIN is also a next-generation electronic medical chart terminal. Because what is seen and heard can be recorded as mobile videos and sounds, respectively, and what is said is automatically recorded through the natural language processing function, the recording times after clinical examinations and interviews are greatly shortened. The medical staff can freely correct the record and add considerations. Fortunately, there is no room for falsification because all records and access logs remain in the artificial neural networks (ANNs) in local medical information centers. If there are "IoT" – compliant communication monitors and printers in the patient's home, and if necessary procedures have been made, the medical staff can easily

Chapter IX

extract the information regarding medical examinations. This IoT infrastructure will be strongly integrated with the environment.

Although it is impossible to monitor the interior of the mind and the contents of thought, it is possible to indirectly fix the psychological state of doctors by monitoring "emotion", "language", and "behavior", because of their exposure to the outside world, together with physical responses.

This is a system expected to bring about calmness and peace of mind from the doctors to the patient at the scene. Specifically, this system monitors the following three points and feeds back their degree of intensity to each doctor as a caution/warning during medical treatment.

> **TON 貪 (greed)**: Monitors feelings of jealousy and urges keeping things close to oneself, among various feelings that occur in medical staff during medical actions.
>
> **JIN 瞋 (rejection and anger)**: Monitors the feelings of anger, irritation, and indifference.
>
> **CHI 痴 (ignoring and laziness)**: Monitors emotions against scientific probability, and laziness based on absolute certainty.

Although the SHIN is embedded with various sensors to monitor the feelings of TON, JIN, and CHI of the medical staff, the SHIN cannot analyze them and give out advice. An artificial neural network server (medical-related ANN-server) that is described in the 技 (GI) analyzes the information and then provides advice. The result of the analysis will be forwarded to the wearable device SHIN instantaneously.

5.2. Multi-agent small type AI/Robot: 技 (GI)

Multi-agent small type AI/Robot 技 (GI) accesses the server of the local medical information center, extracts the medical information of the patient, and displays it (Fig.9-2). A security measure is taken. It is a small-type robot mounted

131

Part 2

with a multi-agent-type AI, and it links to the medical ANNs, which is operated by a regional medical third party and independent committee via a wireless connection. When a patient's personal data is accessed, the patient is immediately informed by the medical information center, and only he or his approved legal representative can access the information.

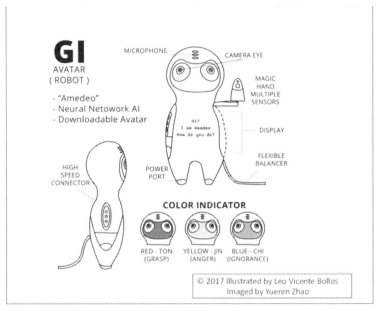

Fig. 9-2: Multi-agent small type AI/Robot: 技 (GI)

Because the cryptographic next-generation block chain technologies are applied, the transparency of the communication of personal information is secured [15]. It is nearly impossible to peek at private information. In the ANNs, a multi-agent type high-performance AI called the "Facilitator AI (FAI)" is assigned to each medical field and sub-specialty. For example, FAI covering general psychiatry and that covering medical care for the elderly are linked together and through the GI that works together with the doctor when he visits a patient at home, they answer the questions that occur at clinical sites.

These AIs converse through an electronic bulletin board called the Black Board; the FAIs take the role of master of ceremonies and lead the others to the optimum solution. The GI – a small-type robot which is smaller than 30 cm in length – is light and can swiftly move and stay near a patient. The robot looks like a cute baby monkey.

The functions of the GI mounted on Amedeo includes constantly monitoring the changes of the three feelings, TON 貪 (greed), JIN 瞋 (rejection and anger), and CHI 痴 (ignoring and laziness). As mentioned earlier, the GI also analyzes the data of the medical staff by relating to the wearable terminal AI function of the SHIN. This is in addition to solving clinical problems through ANNs and communicating at a medical site.

Advice and suggestions are provided to encourage "sharing" in response to the feeling of TON 貪 (greed), "compassion" in response to that of JIN 瞋 (rejecting and anger), and mindfulness in response to CHI 痴 (ignoring and laziness). The functions briefly described in 心 (SHIN) refer to the wisdom of the three detoxification methods of "sharing", "compassion", and "mindfulness" to dispel the three aforementioned problematic emotions.

5.3. Fully-automated general purpose IoT type AI/Robot: 体 (TAI)

"TAI" is a fully-automated vehicle (FAV) – a TAI MODEL MOBILE – whose components are the same as the IoT-type robots. The FAV comes with a mounted lifesaving procedure kit, blood-collection kit and various kinds of automated diagnostic systems applying genetic engineering and patient-oriented self-tracking "life stream" technologies [16]. TAI COCOON BED is a multifunctional bed. It can transform into bed, bathtub, and wheelchair (Fig.9-3).

Part 2

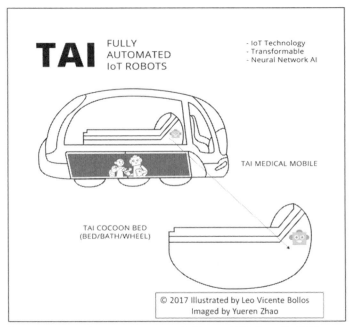

Fig. 9-3: Fully-automated general purpose IoT type AI/Robot 体 (TAI)

6. Applications

The narrative presented below can help one begin to understand transactive relationships among the psychiatrist, the patient, the family, and the Care Robot Trio "SHIN-GI-TAI".

Let's assume that Dr. Ren is a trained physician practicing elderly mental healthcare in collaboration with the Care Robot Trio "SHIN-GI-TAI".

Dr. Ren visits the home of Mr. A (90-year-old, a retired lawyer).

Mr. A has been complaining of insomnia and anxiety, most likely due to fatigue from caring for his partner Mr. B – an 88-year-old retired teacher – who has been lying in bed since a traffic accident that occurred three months ago. So Dr. Ren

Chapter IX

must arrange to go and see Mr. A, and then activate Care Robot Trio "SHIN-GI-TAI" to work with him at the scene.

According to the basic information taken from the local medical information center at the local municipality upon request of a house visit, Mr. A is a former lawyer, living in this community since birth. He lost his parents early and was brought up by his maternal uncle and his wife. He graduated from the local university's law department and got a lawyer qualification at the age of 30. And then, for 40 years, he served the community of social minorities or the causes of socially vulnerable groups, such as advocacy for the welfare of sexual minorities, until he retired at the age of 70. He was 35 when he met Mr. B, a nursery teacher, and he was 50 when they got married.

The couple is childless. Mr. A also has no past medical history of mental or physical illnesses, and his relatives also have no history of mental illness. This was until three months ago, an accident involving the emergency brakes of a MAGLEV bus broke both of his partner's legs.

They usually went to a Go-playing parlor in the community. He opened a free Go class in his own house as an after-school club and he enjoyed teaching Go to several children in the neighborhood three times a week. However, he had stopped holding classes because of the accident.

Dr. Ren is a freelance psychiatrist trained in psychiatric medicine, who worked in a medical corporation with only one physician administrating and providing medical services from 3 to 5 days a week. He received a home visit request from the regional public medical information center in the medical care zone, and so was assigned to be Mr. A's new attending physician for home services.

Dr. Ren's daily work involves contracts with several educational institutes as a part-time child and adolescent psychiatrist at nursery schools, primary schools, junior high schools, high schools, and universities in his community. Along with carrying out mental health services for countermeasures for dementia-related diseases and depression as a family doctor, like in this case, he also performs activities as a school physician. The labor control AI system of the local medical

135

Part 2

information center is used for managing the number of patient activities and actual working hours. Dr. Ren thinks it is the optimal system for psychiatrists to continuously keep their medical facility up to the standard of contemporary medical practices, as opposed to the usual incentive of a high income.

In this visit to Mr. A's house, Dr. Ren booted up the Care Robot Trio "SHIN-GI-TAI", his support device in his daily medical activities at the schools. The Care Robot Trio "SHIN-GI-TAI" belonging to the local emergency physician and Dr. Ren's own "SHIN-GI-TAI" automatically and seamlessly cooperate. Even in Dr. Ren's absence, the emergency physician can respond to emergency home cases based on the patient's latest information. Dr. Ren can visit the patients at their homes immediately, but only in life-threatening cases. These visits happen two or three times a year at most. Then, he visits patients at home riding a fully automated doctor vehicle, or the "TAI".

Dr. Ren carried out a medical examination on Mr. A through an interview regarding his diet, sleep, bowel movements, and daily activity; and then he made a medical examination to obtain brief physical findings including vital signs, pulse check and palpation of the abdomen.

Dr. Ren made the diagnosis that there was no urgent need for a physical examination, and issued an order to release the standby order of TAI MODEL MOBILE type IoT and send it back to the IoT medical base for the use of other medical teams. Dr. Ren ordered Amedeo, who plays the role of the AI-mounted machine GI, to connect with the internal circuit of the bed-type IoT and obtain the information about the care of Mr. B.

Dr. Ren then collected the information on the factors regarding the burden of Mr. A and asked the medical ANN-server to analyze them. The bed-type IoT "TAI" was dispatched to Mr. B. Before Amedeo could connect with its internal circuit, Amedeo first confirmed Mr. B's identity using his individual identification electronic encryption key – which was done by touching the chest portion of the robot. And then the bed-type IoT "TAI" asked Mr. B's approval for what Dr. Ren was about to do for him.

136

Chapter IX

It took only a few minutes to complete Mr. B's approval procedure, to transfer the data to Amedeo from the bed-type TAI, and to complete the analysis at the medical-related server. Amedeo transmitted the result of the analysis to the lens display of Dr. Ren's SHIN in the next room using the wireless function. It was then revealed that Mr. A's care-burden to Mr. B was not that extreme.

After the procedure, Mr. A sat down to talk with Dr. Ren. He told the doctor about his story. He had been living in the region and worked there as a lawyer for many years, and he and his partner have been living humbly and thriving on their communication with the people in the community. Mr. A had not expected his partner to suffer the accident that would render him bedridden. But still he thanked the bed-type robot "TAI", for it helped them maintain their quality of life. And then he said that the reason for his insomnia and anxiety was a common friend. Dr. Ren asked if this friend was elderly as well, but Mr. A replied that she wasn't: it was a little girl in her fourth year of primary school, whom they called C-chan.

When C-chan's mother got remarried last year, Mr. A said, she moved to their region. She often came to the children's club Go class in his house three times a week, together with the other children in the neighborhood. Her mother came home late at night because of her job; C-chan said she did not like to go back home even after the Go class. Mr. A, Mr. B, and C-chan ate supper together and enjoyed their time together until her mother came to pick her up at 10 o'clock. Even after the accident completely debilitated Mr. B, C-chan still came by to see him every day and even helped distract him by playing the Japanese game of 'gomoku-narabe' with him. Three days ago, her stepfather came to pick up C-chan instead of her mother, but C-chan said "I don't want to go back with my step father", and C-chan held on to Mr. B and began to cry.

The bed-type "TAI" recorded video footage of C-chan holding on to Mr. A's partner. Mr. A played the video for Dr. Ren.

Although it was Dr. Ren's mission to hear the elderly man talk about his insomnia and anxiety and find solution, things became a little complicated. It was after this consultation of the couple doing volunteer work in the community that Dr.

137

Part 2

Ren learned the story of a little child in potential danger, whom the couple wanted to protect because of their friendship. Then Mr. B, awakened from his nap, came to the living room from main bedroom together with the bed-type robot "TAI".

He thanked Dr. Ren for coming to the house that day. He asked the doctor if he had heard the story of C-chan from his husband. He said that the little girl came to him while he was bedridden, which she asked him to keep secret; she explained why she was uncomfortable when her stepfather came to pick her up that night. Even though C-chan asked him to keep it a secret, Mr. B decided to divulge what he learned to Mr. A, since he was a lawyer, even though retired, and he felt he could trust him.

What happened was that C-chan happened to be alone with her stepfather while she was taking a nap one day, and she suddenly felt him uncomfortably close to her and then she felt him touching her chest and various parts of her body. C-chan sobbed in terror. Then her stepfather, who had been gentle to her and had never scowled at her before, glowered at her and told her to keep what had happened between the two of them. She must keep it a secret, he said, if she told anybody about it he will make it even worse. C-chan said she didn't tell her mother about it because she didn't want to cause her trouble. Mr. B pleaded for Dr. Ren to help C-chan, and then he wept.

Dr. Ren wanted to help the couple, because of their volunteer work protecting and nurturing children in the regional community. The doctor ordered the AI Amedeo, and the robot GI to analyze the video and he inferred that C-chan's feelings of fear and anger recorded in the video can be relayed to the medical-related ANN-server and there be analyzed.

Dr. Ren did this because he thought that if he compared the information about C-chan with the results from the medical ANNs – which he can access as a school doctor – he could gather more detailed information about C-chan.

However, Dr. Ren didn't expect the response of Amedeo, operating as GI. The robot said:

Chapter IX

"Ren, I understand what you want to do, but we cannot access the information on C-chan. I received a response from the AI of school-related ANNs and it said that if you try to access the information, a notice requiring approval for the provision of information will be sent to her parents, and it will make things complicated. But, if you still want to access it using the access right of a school doctor, you must explain the reason and necessity to the person in charge of the school for you to get approval. I disagree with your plan."

At that time, the 心 (SHIN) monitor sensed Dr. Ren's desire to do a lot of good for the old couple and help C-chan as soon as possible, but it advised that this case is in a state of risk where the feelings "greed", "rejecting and anger" and "ignoring and laziness" intensify. The machine told him: "I advise you to stop your response plan or reconsider it". At the same time, this advice was registered in the FAI of ANNs immediately, which will then become a point of reference in case a similar situation arises in the future. Furthermore, if Dr. Ren agreed with it, the incident report of feeling "greed", "rejecting and anger" and "ignoring and laziness" will be publicized in the third-party committee and others, and then a sort of confession will be taken from him, which will be used as the motivation for behavioral change.

The Care Robot Trio "SHIN-GI-TAI" are servants who observe the instructions of the human responsible for its operation, and at the same time, they are buddies who provide advice and warning to the human. This time also, the SHIN detected Dr. Ren's "suspicious eyes" on Mr. B, a manifestation of the feeling of rejection and anger which occurred in the doctor's mind, which passed for a moment as a look on his face, and the medical-related ANN-server analyzed it as "rejection and anger" and then was instantaneously linked to the Avatar Robot GI (here Amedeo is GI) and the SHIN of Amedeo, and the robots provided Dr. Ren the advice with which to trigger the feeling of tenderness for other person.

Dr. Ren is familiar with the SHIN named "Amedeo" and treats its AI as a buddy. Amedeo will continue to monitor and encourage the doctor – whose body and mind are continually deteriorating – until his retirement at age 70.

139

Part 2

7. Discussion

7.1. The SHIN and medical ANNs did not overlook the doctor's facial expression

Receiving the information from medical ANNs, Amedeo called Dr. Ren via earphone by his nickname. The AI said: "Ren, Mr. A and Mr. B are pioneers of same-sex marriage. You had better ask them directly in detail". Basically, Amedeo does not possess loudspeakers that would allow him to communicate to other people simultaneously. He can only communicate to one person – which in this case is Dr. Ren – the minimum necessary information through the wireless earphone of the 心 (SHIN) device.

Protecting the "individual dignity" of patients and medical staff, medical ANNs monitor the feelings of "greed", "rejection and anger" and "ignoring and laziness", and at the same time, the ANNs monitor the principles of mental healthcare and the moral hazards relating to medical ethics and the possible biases of the medical staff themselves. The system is run such that medical staff can always do self-reflection, so that their feelings and their words and behavior do not undermine their personal dignity.

The wisdom of Theravada Buddhism can be seen in the algorithm enabling the systems of SHIN, GI and TAI to provide advice when the problematic feelings "greed", "rejection and anger" and "ignoring and laziness" occur in the medical staff. The greatest care is required to protect children's rights. However, the AI network summarized its opinion that using the access right of the school doctor in that situation would have brought about the opposite effect. Yet it is also Dr. Ren's judgment and responsibility as clinical doctor to do his best to provide the best solution to the problem faced by Mr. A, Mr. B, and C-chan.

Dr. Ren advised them that the best way to help C-chan would be for Mr. B – who received C-chan's admission of molestation – to visit the appropriate counter at child welfare together with Mr. A, the lawyer, and ask for a coping scheme for C-chan. The doctor also told them that he would accompany them there as the

140

Chapter IX

attending doctor of Mr. B, and he would support them so that they can have calm judgment and behavior.

Mr. B thanked the doctor for his help. He requested Dr. Ren to place their conversation about C-chan onto the official record and restrict C-chan's access to it. The doctor promised to make the necessary arrangements immediately. He also said he would include self-reflection in the records.

Dr. Ren promised to visit Mr. B for a medical examination, again, after a week. Mr. A said to him when he was leaving that he and his partner are going to a Go parlor soon, though without the bed-type IoT care robot, he couldn't get down from the 10th floor of his apartment.

Dr. Ren registered all records of the day's medical examination into the ANNs, designating them as restricted information, and then he issued the instruction to report that a specific child's rights were threatened (possibility of child abuse) to a medical information center, revealing himself – a care physician – to be the source of the information.

7.2. Human-to-intelligent machine are artificial relationships and technology-dependent, while transactive relationships are guided by ethics

Isaac Asimov proposed the "Three Laws of Robotics" in 1950 [17] as the three fundamental principles that robots must comply with so they could contribute to human beings and so eliminate the possibility of uncontrolled robots in the process. These rules are:

1) A robot may not injure a human being or, through inaction, allow a human being to come to harm.

2) A robot must obey orders given it by human beings except where such orders would conflict with the First Law.

3) A robot must protect its own existence as long as such protection does not conflict with the First or Second Law.

141

Part 2

7.3. New five laws for care robots user (The "I" declaration)

It is presumed that it will be necessary to address various new ethical tasks for the AI robots in the world by 2035 to 2050, including tasks regarding the three fundamental principles that robots will not be able to cope with, especially the protection of private information and concerns for lives other than those of human beings.

Thus, the authors proposed the New Five Laws for Care Robot Users to live meaningful and healthy lives with the help of Care Robots, relating to the Buddhist Five Precepts (pañca-sila) [18].

7.3.1. Article 1 【Abandoning the taking of life】
I undertake the precept to refrain from destroying living creatures using Care Robots.

Prohibition of the use of military robots for care purposes and prohibition of the use of Care Robots for military purposes.

Article 1 proclaims that Care Robots must not hurt or kill not only human beings but also all other beings and creatures. This article forces developers, operators, and sellers to comply with the fundamental principles respecting the dignity of life. Therefore, the military robots which are programmed to end life should not be repurposed as Care Robots, and Care Robots should not be diverted to military support. Furthermore, the individuals, organizations, and companies responsible for the development, operation, and sales of Care Robots should not have conflicts of interest with military officials, military organizations, or military industries.

7.3.2. Article 2 【Abandoning stealing】
I undertake the precept to refrain from taking that which is not given using Care Robots.

Article 2 clearly specifies that Care Robots should not be used as a tool for stealing others' tangible and intangible assets and information.

142

Chapter IX

7.3.3. Article 3 【Abandoning illicit sex】
I undertake the precept to refrain from sexual misconduct using Care Robots.

Article 3 orders users of robots not to intrude on privacy, threaten the dignity of individuals, as well as not to perform socially deviant actions, including economic and sexual exploitation. It also prohibits information manipulation and cover-ups by business operators of Care Robots, communications and information technology companies, and the authorities concerned. Care Robots must be used only under the right program distributed to the site by the development, management, and sales departments of robot manufacturers through a transparent and open process.

7.3.4. Article 4 【Abandoning lying】
I undertake the precept to refrain from incorrect speech using Care Robots. I do not incorporate programs and algorithms for such applications into Care Robots.

Article 4 instructs providers, owners and users not to deceive other people using Care Robots or use them to disturb the harmony of other people.

7.3.5. Article 5 【Abandoning the use of intoxicants】
I undertake the precept to refrain from intoxicating drinks and drugs which can lead to carelessness, while I develop, operate, and instruct Care Robots programs.

Article 5 promulgates the necessary basic safety knowledge which the developers of Care Robots should always observe, such as avoiding operating the robots or directing people to use the robots under the influence of psychotropic substances.

143

Part 2

8. Conclusion

The virtual caring situation is a blueprint for the upcoming prediction that the "encounter between people" included in this situation will revolve around the elements of caring and its ethical issues by 2050. The authors have provided a description of possible future care that follows the precepts of Buddhist thought, rather than the Western ways the medical community had been used to observing.

This chapter projected possible human caring from the viewpoint of transactive relations facilitated by the use of Care Robots. It is speculated that in the future, the environments of virtual reality and the actual reality will come to exist together. Also, this chapter considered the benefits and risks of scientific and technological progress that can occur around the future patient (region, environment, people, etc.) which might affect his care.

References

[1] Kelly K: THE ENEVITABLE – Understanding the 12 Technological Forces That Will Shape Our Future, [Kindle version_2]. Introduction, para 19. Retrieved from Amazon.com 3. 2016.

[2] Arai H, Ouchi Y, Toba K, et al.: Japan as the front-runner of super-aged societies: Perspectives from medicine and medical care in Japan. Geriatr Gerontol Int, Vol. 15, No. 6, pp. 673-87, 2015. DOI: 10.1111/ggi.12450. Epub 2015 Feb 5.

[3] Charlotte B, Shirley G, Beth K (Eds): Nursing Case Studies in Caring: Across the Practice Spectrum 1st Edition, Springer Publishing Company, 2015.

[4] Tanioka T: The Development of the Transactive Relationship Theory of Nursing (TRETON): A Nursing Engagement Model for persons and Robots and Humanoid Nursing Robots. Int J Nurs Clin Pract, Vol. 4, IJNCP-223, 2017.
DOI: 10.15344/2394-4978/2017/223

[5] "Purification of Mind", by Bhikkhu Bodhi. Access to Insight (Legacy Edition), 5 June 2010
http://www.accesstoinsight.org/lib/authors/bodhi/bps-essay_04.html

144

Chapter IX

[6] "Mula Sutta: Roots" (AN 3.69), translated from the Pali by Thanissaro Bhikkhu. Access to Insight (Legacy Edition), 3 July 2010. http://www.accesstoinsight.org/tipitaka/an/an03/an03.069.than.html.

[7] Kelly K: THE ENEVITABLE – Understanding the 12 Technological Forces That Will Shape Our Future, [Kindle version_2]. Introduction, para 19. Retrieved from Amazon.com, 2016.

[8] Arai H, Ouchi Y, Yokode M, Ito H, et al.: Toward the realization of a better aged society: Messages from gerontology and geriatrics. Geriatrics & Gerontology International, Vol. 12, No. 1, pp. 16-22, 2012. DOI: 10.1111/j.1447-0594.2011.00776.x

[9] Kurzweil R, Grossman T: Fantastic voyage: live long enough to live forever. The science behind radical life extension questions and answers. Stud Health Technol Inform, Vol. 149, pp. 187-194, 2009. DOI: 10.3233/978-1-60750-050-6-187

[10] Gray AJ: Stigma in psychiatry. Journal of the Royal Society of Medicine, Vol. 95, No. 2, pp.72-76, 2002.

[11] Corrigan PW, Watson AC: Understanding the impact of stigma on people with mental illness. World Psychiatry, Vol. 1, No. 1, pp. 16-20, 2002.

[12] Shrivastava A, Johnston M, Bureau Y: Stigma of Mental Illness-1: Clinical reflections. Mens Sana Monographs, Vol. 10, No. 1, pp. 70-84, 2012. DOI:10.4103/0973-1229.90181

[13] Vos R, Houtepen R, Horstman K: Evidence-based medicine and power shifts in health care systems. Health Care Anal, Vol. 10, No. 3, pp. 319-28, 2002.

[14] Moira Stewart, Brian W Gilbert: Reflections on the doctor–patient relationship: from evidence and experience. Br J Gen Pract, Vol. 55, No. 519, pp. 793–801, 2005.

[15] Dean C: How Many Bitcoin Are Mined Per Day? Bitcoin Stack Exchange. March 28, 2013.

[16] Carreiro N, Fertig S, Freeman E, et al.: Lifestreams: Bigger Than Elvis. Yale University, March 25, 1996.

145

Part 2

[17] Asimov I: I, Robot, 1950.

[18] Access to Insight: The Five Precepts: pañca-sila.
http://www.accesstoinsight.org/ptf/dhamma/sila/pancasila.html
(Accessed 30 November 2013)

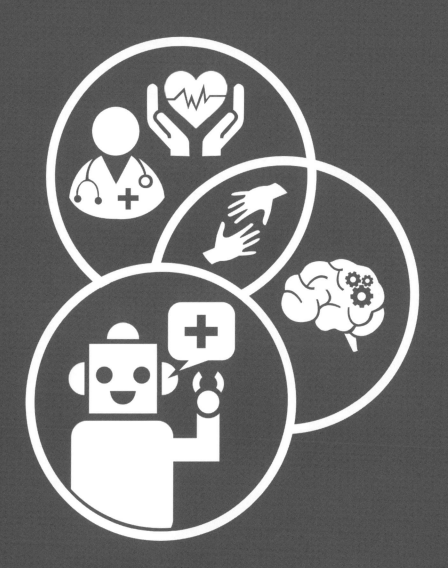

PART 03

The possibility of relating in nursing, technologies in healthcare, caring, humanoid nurse robots, artificial intelligence, and corresponding health issues.

© 2017 Illustrated by Leo Vicente Bollos

Part 3

Abstract

This chapter engages in a critical examination of this emergence and asks what the role of robotics should be in nursing and, more broadly, what implications emerge for patients and the nursing profession. The future of nursing in Western and other wealthy countries is predicted to be linked strongly with automated robotics for efficient and cost-effective care. Their emergence and predicted roles are associated strongly with care of the body and more broadly with communicating with and assisting people with their daily living activities.

Key Words: Healthcare, Robotics, Nursing, Technology, Activities of daily living, Patient-centered care

Chapter X

A Critical Examination of Robotics

and the Sacred in Nursing

By Alan Barnard

Chapter X

1. Introduction

Nurses have always used technology, and the emergence of robots in nursing practice introduces another part of the journey of development – a journey which will be a radical detour for us as we begin to see the emergence of a new and probable independent contributor to direct care. It will be radical because rather than being a passive technology that we use for organizing our individual practice, data collection, and measuring body function and metrics, robots will potentially have an independent and proactive role in healthcare delivery. Eventually automated robots will make independent decisions and initiate delivery of nursing care, sometimes without a human presence [1-4].

The inclusion of automated robotics in nursing is a whole new level of technology engagement for nursing, especially since so much of the projected roles for robots is associated with embodied activities that have been central to nursing practice and the maintenance of activities of daily living (ADL). Body care activities have included lifting people, assisting patients to walk, assisting patients with toileting, cleaning the body, feeding people, and engaging in supportive communication. These are the types of activities that by their very nature have been sacred to nursing as core elements of practice, theory, skills, knowledge, and professional responsibility in healthcare [5-8]. For example, in Dorothea Orem's self-care deficit theory [9], nursing care is necessary when a person is unable to fulfill identified biological, psychological, developmental, or social needs. Orem's theory emphasizes the needs of the person and their body, as a fundamental core element of nursing as a discipline. In clinical practice our responsibility includes managing care of the body and the associated activities are central to the modern nursing role [5]. Although literature has tended to trivialize activities such as caring for the body as gendered, and stereotype women (who have been associated commonly with these activities) as technologically incapable and ignorant [10], we see now in robotics an interest in body care, and more broadly the efficient provision of activities of daily living through the intervention of robots. Suddenly the body has

149

Part 3

become far more important to people outside of nursing. The development of robotics is bringing a whole new appreciation for body care, and robotics is emerging as the way to solve emerging human resource restrictions as populations age and a new frontier for economic profit.

This chapter examines robotics in relation to this new appreciation and from a second order perspective. That is, rather than being concerned about the efficiency of procedures that can be achieved with robots, or their best design, this chapter asks: What should be the relation between robotics, nursing practice and person-focused care?

2. Robots are the answer, but what was the question?

People have a right to great quality healthcare, and meeting the health needs of people is at the very core of nursing practice. Even though nursing is more than physical care, so much of our practice involves technology and we do tend to focus on the practical potential of technology, but not the implications for our roles. Sharts-Hopco [3] noted that despite predictions that the healthcare robotics industry will reach a value of 50 billion US dollars by 2025, and there is already an explosion of developmental work on personal care robotics especially in Japan [11], the author identified only one relevant article from nursing in the international literature related to discussion of the profound changes and challenges robotics will bring to nursing. This situation occurs also even though unpredictability has been identified regularly as a central feature of technological progress [12, 13]. Good use of technology requires early and ongoing assessment of likely effects for people, nurses, and the profession; that is, assessment to the best of our ability. But a chronic lack of engagement and more broad thinking about the effects of technology on care will hinder robotics from becoming optimal contributors to healthcare across the range of contexts. Robotics in aged care alone are predicted to revolutionize the industry; it is an industry dominated by nurses and nurse assistance and is growing worldwide [11].

150

Chapter X

Automated robotics will require alteration to scope of practice, governance of care, policies, organizational systems, and the professional cultures that determine information and resources. Predictions about the size and breadth of change are not just about fear of redundancy (that is, fear of nurses being replaced by robots), but of equal importance is the need for reflection on developments in robotics and what they can bring to nursing and healthcare [11]. Unsurprisingly, the International Organization for Standardization (ISO) recently developed ISO 13482 which is aimed at protecting organizations against litigation [14]. Their focus is on encouraging close robot interaction but with protections against any unforeseen accidents. The standard is about ensuring care robots and humans remain safe, and Daniella Muoio highlights three categories of robotic assistance that the ISO standard is seeking to address: physical assistant robots, mobile servant robots, and person carrier robots [15].

Nurse leaders need to plan now for leading the integration of robotics into the many domains of nursing, not simply waiting to respond to their presence. Nursing has a history of acceptance of technology without critical examination. Repetition of this behavior, for example, will not be useful and may lead to attitudes expressed by Whyatt who cited an assistant Head of Nursing in the UK who believed that even if clinical nursing care is delivered by robots, "ultimately health managers will decide whether or not a robot can do a nurse's job" (p.67) [16]. Responsibility for the future of nursing practice and healthcare must involve more than robots doing nursing work, and acceptance of change is a logical aspiration. The degree of adaptation necessary in order for nurses to maintain person-focused care and participate as leaders will be enormous, and the implications even bigger.

Evidence is clear as to the influence of technologies on behavior(s) and professions. Witness for example the influence of computers and the internet on each person. Langdon Winner highlighted 40 years ago that technological innovation influences every aspect of a society (and professional group) [17]. Customs, values, ideas, language, behavior, attitudes, etc. are changed often to accommodate change. Actions must alter, customs and practices must give way to

151

Part 3

new ideas, and sometimes long-held values must be rejected in preference for new perspectives. Whilst some change to nursing practice will bring improvement, ignorance of the full extent and influence of technological development from the field of robotics on the nursing profession is challenging. However, it is unfortunate that there is little debate to inform understanding and reflection at a time when more is needed to inform nurses of unanswered questions concerning robotics and nursing.

3. Nurses and robots

There have been important periods of technological change in nursing over the past 50 years. From 1965-80 greater automated technology and the emergence of specialization emerged, and from 1980-90 increased technical control, streamlined care, automated devices and monitoring equipment all emerged. A further, more recent period of change has seen rapid information access and retrieval and the emergence of care delivery at a distance [18-20].

We now see in wealthy Western countries the use of integrated healthcare records, decision support software, wearable monitors, smart phone applications, and the early emergence of robot-assisted care delivery [21]. Importantly, robots have a number of key features that define their status as a "robot", which include the ability to make autonomous decisions and operate in real world environments without external control. A robot by definition brings with it an ability to act on the world as if it can "think" and be autonomous. That is to say, a robot must have some degree of autonomy and be "situated in the world" as an actor within it. A computer is not a robot as it cannot make autonomous decisions based on thinking, nor can it initiate actions on its own behalf to bring about a non-predefined outcome. Computers are involved in the design and functioning of a robot, but a robot brings with it much greater self-determination, responsibility, unpredictability, and volition. It is predicted that robots will become increasingly self-determinate, able to initiate care through their own will, learn from mistakes, and exhibit some degree of

152

designed emotional and intellectual engagement; we will soon start to talk about nurse and patient, and robot and patient care [11, 22].

Robots will be under the direction of someone (possibly a nurse), but will have a degree of independence in a broader healthcare environment. Already there is increasing application of robotics in nursing contexts. There are companionship robots such as JustoCat and PARO the therapeutic seal and robots that transport resources (e.g. pharmaceuticals) (HelpMate), that pick up and place people into bed (Care-O-Bot; RI-MAN), that provide education and verbal guidance, give encouragement (Nurse-Bot), and feed people (MY SPOON) [1, 11, 23-28].

These and similar robotic devices do not fully fulfil a strict definition of robot, but represent early developments that foreshadow the shape of things to come very quickly onto the healthcare scene. There are many potential robot applications including cleaning, feeding patients, preparing food, attending to an emergency, bathing, responding to emotional stimuli, administering medication, walking patients, driving a car, and guiding people as they walk around [3]. Many of these activities are nursing task-related and robot involvement will impact directly on nursing practice.

4. Robots and the sacred in nursing

Although principally an automated device like all technology(ies), robots will change the very nature of nursing practice, the institutions we work in, the conceptual frameworks we use for the nursing profession, and the ideas we have about safety and comfort [29, 30]. Practice methods will change, scope of practice will evolve, and current assumptions about caring will need to be (re)examined.

We have typically tended to focus on robotics in terms of the reaction(s) humans have to robots; that is, how humans react to robot technology. The uncanny valley experiments [31] are an example of seeking to know the association between robots, emotion, and acceptance; it seems that if a robot looks too much like a human we struggle to accept them. Although this work is important, in nursing,

Part 3

however, we need to consider the reverse of this commonplace [29]. Robots have been proposed as a potential source of empathetic support for patients. Nurses already work as partners with robots in the provision of care, especially in the aged care sector(s) [1, 11, 26, 32]. Robotic applications are increasing rapidly in breadth and scope, and eventually patients will primarily communicate with an autonomous personal robot who will provide care; that is, sometimes a human nurse may not always communicate directly with the patient about an issue or problem.

This issue is a crucial factor for nursing and healthcare provision, since as a constructed phenomenon, robots do not have a knowingness; that is, robots will never have a consciousness as you and I would understand it. In the future a robot may be able to express an emotional response as a predetermined protocol/reaction, but a robot will not understand emotion in a human sense, and know compassion in the same way. Importantly, it is at this axis point that human nurses must seek to maintain position, uniqueness, and contribution [33]. It is likely robots will be able to accomplish with greater accuracy nearly all aspects of care we currently provide, but it is at the level of the personal that robotics will struggle and it is where human nurses must demonstrate their importance. Robots will achieve proficiency in repetitive jobs, administrative roles, automated responsibilities, and the preparation and provision of pre-defined interventions. Contrary to popular nursing literature, such as the blog "The truth about nursing [34]", robots will for example achieve the ability to inform a physician of an incorrect treatment, wrong operation, and an incorrect patient. They will be able to call security, contact and coordinate members of the multidisciplinary team, and when required assess patients on presentation to an emergency ward. But what they won't do well is adequately deal with irrational, emotional, and unpredictable human responses and behavior.

Interestingly, what engenders the most enthusiasm about robotics often is their potential to usefully undertake menial activity-(-ies), but of equal importance is the goal to create an illusion of intelligence. However, despite advances in cognition, automation, and automated autonomous action, Bekey notes [35] that robots struggle to achieve the ability to make meaningful personal human-to-human connection.

154

Chapter X

The specifics of their action and behaviors fail dramatically when attempting to engage in subjective and emotional connection with a human. For example, although a robot can dispense pharmaceutics, it will not for example, deal well with anger and frustration when expressed by a patient, except to call for assistance, and may struggle to prioritize important conflicting demands related to acute illness or emergency [35]. Feelings of frustration leading to emotions such as anger can often appear irrational and seemingly inappropriate to the causes of human reaction in scale or intensity. It is therefore not surprising to note that Metzler, Lewisy, and Pope [33] highlight that robotics developers struggle with these aspects of human interaction; in particular, creating the illusion in robotics that they can mimic human concern and interaction. Ultimately Turkle [36] notes, a robot does not have any level of phenomenological engagement (life consciousness) in terms of personal knowing and will always risk failure in the area of human connection and relationships.

It is a fact that robots struggle with the depth of human personal and subjective experience and connection and will continue to do so [37]. Recognition of emotional expression is achievable, but that success is only a small part of the puzzle that makes up human interaction and communication. Understanding the reasons behind our patients' reactions to the dispensing of pharmaceutics and their associated anger and frustration (as an example of the broader issue of human connection) is a significant problem and will be a clinical void that human nurses will need to fill. The reasons for feelings and emotions can be complex and a daunting challenge for any robot, especially when considering that even humans can struggle with this type of engagement. For example, our patient's anger could be caused by perceived failure of a doctor to visit the person, and the patient transfers their frustration and resultant anger onto the robot during medication administration; their anger was really about their care.

Nonetheless the potential for robots as major contributors in aged care and for mild dementia through interventions such as robot pet therapy (PARO therapeutic baby seal robot) is demonstrated as a focus in robotics development [27, 32, 38].

155

Part 3

Currently robots act in the world through behavior and sound, often in response to touch and voice. They demonstrate some therapeutic effects in assisting agitated people in conditions such as dementia [32]. At a solely instrumental level, many of the physical activities of a care giver can (will) be replicated by robots; physical assistance can be provided without knowing or feeling empathy, or engaging in the development of a human relationship. At one level the work and business of healthcare provision can get done, but nursing care is supposed to be much more than that; it is a human-centric activity grounded to some degree within connection at a personal and subjective level [4, 16].

It is not surprising to note therefore that sentience is the ultimate goal of robotic development. That is, the ability to create the illusion of an ability/capacity to perceive and experience subjectivity (to be able to think and evaluate individual experience and thought). Borenstein and Pearson [37] speculate that there remains widespread uncertainty as to the effect of robots on human relations, because of the very nature of their emergence. Even though it is noted that humans in Western culture do tend to nurture computers and other objects [39], often forming close bond and association (e.g. ownership of an automobile can include giving the object a name and worrying about its welfare), robot sentience (no matter how clever it becomes) will remain an illusion, since a robot can never achieve its own existential presence – a robot is not born into a world of human caring and connection; a robot is placed within it [33, 36].

But even with this deficit, could experiences with robots be characterized as meaningful enough to create a sense of interest and concern? Borenstein and Pearson [37] emphasize that robot reactions to human behavior and emotions may be more important than their appearance when caring for people and seeking to gain patient acceptance. Responding physically in ways that give an appearance of understanding and empathy appear to be key criteria for success, noting importantly that distinctions in care provision need to be drawn between shallow, deep and good care, when provided by a robot [40]. Shallow care refers to care provided in an instrumental fashion that lacks intimacy, engagement on a personal level, or

Chapter X

evidence of emotional connection and communication. Good care is described as having respect for human dignity, and importantly for robotic assistance, deep care is grounded in reciprocity and a depth of mutual understanding of feelings and emotions. Robots will not achieve deep care in their role, certainly not until they can genuinely feel emotions expressed as genuine sorrow, love or despair.

The outcomes for human relations are speculative, and we have not decided what kind of patient care a robot should deliver. But in their defense is this question: Is a robot who provides physical care well any less genuine than a human nurse who does not feel and express any empathy? Would lack of concern by a human nurse who practices based on scripted communication, protocols, and constructed emotional support [41] be any more or less a positive experience than care provided by an automated robot? If an impression of understanding, caring, and companionship is all that is needed, then a robot may be an excellent and viable option in care delivery.

5. Robots and the illusion of neutrality

Winner [42] confirmed a characterization of many authors, most notably Engels, that when technology develops so do social environments and hierarchies of control which are required to keep participants acting in a desired manner. The term 'required' in this case is understood in a practical sense and is important for nurses. Nursing as a discipline is part of this emerging contexts of change, and risks being enveloped by innovations in this area and potentially devalued through robotics. Who needs a human nurse for practical tasks when the same task could be effectively and efficiently completed by an autonomous robot? Further to this, as an agent of action an autonomous robot providing care to another person reproduces nursing values and norms through its actions, behaviors and responses. Their quality of nursing care will reflect on human nurses, since as providers of care they will produce moral action(s) (that is, through their care robots will make clinical decisions about choice and suitability of care). Robots will be representatives of the

157

Part 3

broader nursing profession [43], and they must be able to act and function in ways that raise the profession in all aspects of their practice. If they cannot, robots will not make a useful contribution to nursing and healthcare.

People have a right to high quality nursing care, and even though technology will often assist in this goal, by virtue of our professional role(s) we should be responsible for effectively utilizing and integrating appropriate technology, including robots, in the provision of that care. Almerud, et al. [44] argue that every nurse faces the challenge to provide care with the assistance of technology, but at the same time, positively contribute to the patients' lived experience. They highlight the ambiguity this presents for nurses in the use of technology, because embracing human-centered care and technical proficiency are not necessarily the same thing.

Current discussions in nursing (the emphasis is on discussion since there is still limited debate) require serious reflection, because observations mirror what has so often been the tenet of nursing literature related to technology; i.e. excitement about embracing technology [45]. The American Sentinel [46] noted that as robots become more autonomous and agile, and available to assist through an emerging nursing shortage, healthcare organizations will seek to use robots in selected nursing roles, adding further that nurse leaders will be required to ensure that "high-tech" does not replace the "high-touch". The observation is most likely correct, but the level of naiveté and willingness of the author to simply hand over to robotics what will be many of the fundamental aspects of nursing care delivery associated with ADL's, without detailed and earnest examination of implications and effects for patients and care more broadly, is astounding.

Efficiency, precision, productivity, resource management, and technological progress appear to be ends in themselves, and achieving professional and moral ideals which in nursing relate often to human-centered practices will in reality become increasingly less likely. Schon [13] identified three effects of technological progress; the desired, the foreseen, and the unforeseen. Each effect cannot be fully predicted, and it was demonstrated clearly that the inclusion of technology in contexts of clinical practice alters the practice of nurses [45, 47]. Technology will to

158

a greater or lesser extent influence a nurse's capacity to accomplish practice goals, display caring behaviors, and maintain principles of practice, particularly when it is governed by policy, work overload, high acuity patients, and limited resources.

Robots will not be a neutral addition to the ways nurses care for people on a daily basis. Robotics will influence consideration of culture, spirituality, emotional connection, and physical care [4, 20, 43, 48-50]. Robots like any technology will not lead always to treatment outcomes acceptable for patients, but will not be an influence that leads always to uncaring inhospitable wards. Robots have potential to assist healthcare outcomes across a range of possibilities from positive to negative within holistic frameworks with awareness and planning [30], but the centrality of the person and by extension their values, choices and individual experiences will be the measure of success.

Some nurses appear prepared already to hand over nursing care associated with assistance with daily living to robotics for the promise of technological advancement as if it is a fair exchange; it is not. The costs to professional independence, self-determination, and changes to patient care will be momentous and will need serious consideration and debate.

6. Conclusion

Robotics will be a major contributor to changing healthcare systems in developed countries. They will influence the way we live our lives, nursing practice, and the experience(s) of healthcare. The inclusion of robotics in care provision will be transformative and their presence will alter the way(s) we practice on a daily basis. The growth of robotics will lead to enormous advances that will be important, exciting and at the same time challenging. It is therefore very likely that new approaches to nursing practice will be required to maximize robotic involvement, while at the same time, ensuring we are responsive to the specifics of human experience [51]. The advantages of robotics and the many changes they will bring to healthcare and nursing care will need to be balanced with an ongoing struggle for a

Part 3

humane and caring healthcare system(s). Productive critique is required that seeks ways for nurses to lead and respond appropriately to robotics as an important future development in healthcare provision and human relations. What will make nursing responsive to changing contexts will be emphasizing that assistance with daily living is a foundation of nursing care provision, is central to human needs, is a determining factor in the quality of healthcare, and is inseparable from the control of nursing. The areas of concern and interest raised in this chapter need serious discussion and debate. They have direct relationship to your future as a nurse because good planning and appropriate integration of robotics will be important in future care for your patients.

References

[1] Broadbent E, Kerse N, Peri K, Robinson H, et al.: Benefits and problems of health-care robots in aged care settings: A comparison trial. Australasion Journal of Ageing, Vol. 35, pp. 23-29, 2016. DOI: 10.1111/ajag.12190

[2] Robinson H, Macdonald B, Kerse N, Broadbent E: Suitability of healthcare robots for a dementia unit and suggested improvements. JAMDA, Vol. 14, pp. 34-40, 2013. DOI: 10.1016/j.jamda.2012.09.006

[3] Sharts-Hopko N: The coming revolution in personal care robotics. What does it mean for nurses? Nursing Adminstration, Vol. 38, pp. 5-12, 2014. DOI: 10.1097/NAQ.0000000000000000

[4] Wynsberghe AV: Designing robots for care: Care centred value-sensitive design. Sci Eng Ethics, Vol. 19, pp. 407-433, 2013. DOI: 10.1007/s11948-011-9343-6

[5] Draper J: Embodied practice: rediscovering the 'heart' of nursing. Journal of Advanced Nursing, Vol. 70, pp. 2235-2244, 2014. DOI: 10.1111/jan.12406

[6] George J: Nursing theories: the base for professional nursing practice (6th Ed). Pearson, 2014.

[7] Henderson V: The Nature of Nursing: A Definition and its Implications for Practice, Research, and Education. New York, Macmillan Publishing, 1966.

Chapter X

[8] Sakalys JA: Bringing Bodies Back In: Embodiment and Caring Science. International Journal for Human Caring, Vol. 10, pp. 17-21, 2006. DOI: 106348525

[9] Orem D: Nursing: Concepts and practice (6th Ed). St. Louis, MO: Mosby, 2001.

[10] Wajcman J: Feminism Confronts Technology. Polity Press, Cambridge, 1991.

[11] Ross A: The industries of the future. Simon and Schuster, London, 2016.

[12] Ellul J: The technological bluff. Eerdmans, Michigan, 1990.

[13] Schon D: Technology and change; the impact of invention and innovation on American social and economic development. Delta, New York, 1967.

[14] International Organisation of Standardisation 2014 Robots and robotic devices – Safety requirements for personal care robots ISO13482:2014.

http://www.iso.org/iso/catalogue_detail?csnumber=53820

(Accessed 10 November 2016)

[15] Japan is running out of people to take care of the elderly, so it's making robots instead.

http://www.businessinsider.com.au/japan-developing-carebots-for-elderly-care-201

5-11?r=US&IR=T: (Accessed 17 October 2016)

[16] Whyatt J: Could a robot do your job? Nursing Standard, Vol. 28, pp. 66-6, 2014. DOI: 10.7748/ns2014.04.28.34.66.s50

[17] Winner L: Autonomous technology. MIT Press, Massachusett, 1977.

[18] Barnard A, Sinclair M: Spectators and spectacles: nurses, midwives and visuality. Journal of Advanced Nursing Vol. 55, pp. 578-586, 2006. DOI: 10.1111/j.1365-2648.2006.03947.x

[19] Rinard R: Technology, deskilling, and nurses: the impact of the technologically changing environment. Advances in Nursing Science, Vol. 18, pp. 60-70, 1996. DOI: 00012272-199606000-00008

[20] Sandelowski M: Devices and desires: gender, technology and American nursing. University of North Carolina, Chapel Hill, 2000.

[21] Monteiro A: Cyborgs, biotechnologies, and Informatics In health care – new paradigms in nursing science. Nursing Philosophy, Vol. 17, No. 1, pp. 19-27, 2016. DOI: 10.1111/nup.12088

161

Part 3

[22] THE CONVERSATION: Robots in healthcare could lead to a doctorless hospital. http://theconversation.com/robots-in-health-care-could-lead-to-a-doctorless-hospital-54316 (Accessed 21 November 2016)

[23] Beedholm K, Frederiksen K, Skovsgaard Frederiksen A, Lomborg K: Attitudes to a robot bathtub in Danish elder care: A hermeneutic study. Nursing and Health Sciences, Vol. 17, pp. 280-286, 2015. DOI: 10.1111/nhs.12184

[24] Gerling K, Hebesberger D, Dondrup C, Kortner T, Hanheide M: Robot deployment in long term care. Zeitschriftt fur Gerontologie und Geriatrie, Vol. 49, pp. 288-297, 2016. DOI: 10.1007/s00391-016-1065-6

[25] Banks M, Willoughby L, Banks W: Animal-assisted therapy and loneliness in nursing homes: Use of robotic versus living dogs. JAMDA, Vol. 3, pp.173-177, 2008. DOI: 10.1016/j.jamda.2007.11.007

[26] Joranson N, Pedersen I, Rokstad A, Ihlebaek C: Effects on symptoms of agitation and depression in persons with dementia participating in robot-assisted activity: A cluster-randomised controlled trial. JAMDA, Vol. 16, pp. 867-873, 2015.
DOI: 10.1016/j.jamda.2015.05.002

[27] Joranson N, Pedersen I, Rokstad A, Aamodt G, Olsen C, Ihlebaek C: Group activity with Paro in nursing homes: systematic investigation of behaviors in participants. International psychogeriatrics, Vol. 28, pp. 1345-1354, 2016.
DOI: 10.1017/s1041610216000120

[28] Robinson H, Broadbent E: Group sessions with PARO in a nursing home: Structure, observation and interviews. Australasian Journal of Ageing, Vol. 35 pp. 106-112, 2016. DOI: 10.1111/ajag.12199

[29] Erikson H, Salzmann-Erikson M: Future challenges of robotics and artificial intelligence in nursing: What can we learn from monsters in popular culture? The Permanente Journal, Vol. 20, pp. 15-243, 2016. DOI: 10.7812/TPP/15-243

[30] Fuji S, Ito H, Yasuhara Y, Huang S, Tanioka T, Locsin RC: Discussion of Nursing Robot's Capability and Ethical Issues. Proceedings of 2014 INFORMATION, Vol. 17, No. 1, pp. 349-353, 2014.

[31] Mori M: The uncanny valley.

Chapter X

http://spectrum.ieee.org/automaton/robotics/humanoids/the-uncanny-valley
(Accessed 24 November 2016)

[32] Soler M, Aguera_Ortiz L, Rodriguez J, et al.: Social robots in advanced dementia. Frontiers in aging neuroscience, Vol. 7, pp. 1-12, 2015.
DOI: 10.3389/fnagi.2015.00133

[33] Metzler TA, Lewis LM, Pope LC: Could robots become authentic companions in nursing care? Nursing Philosophy, Vol. 17, pp. 36-48, 2016.
DOI: 10.1111/nup.12101

[34] THE TRUTH ABOUT NURSING: Can Robots be Nurses?
https://www.truthaboutnursing.org/faq/robonurse.html (Accessed 20 October 2016)

[35] Bekey GA: Current trends in robotics. In: Lin P, Abney K, Bekey GA (Eds). Robot ethics: The ethical and social implications of robotics. MIT Press, Massachusetts, pp. 17-24, 2012.

[36] Turkle S: Alone together: why we expect more from technology and less from each other. Basic Books, New York, 2011.

[37] Borenstein J, Pearson Y: Robot caregivers: ethical issues across the human lifespan. In: Lin P, Abney K, Bekey GA (Eds) Robot Ethics: The ethical and social implications of robots. MIT Press, Massachusetts, pp. 251-265, 2012.

[38] Mesquita A, Zamarioli C, Carvalho E: The use of robots in nursing care practices: an explorative-descriptive study. Online Brazilian Journal of Nursing, Vol. 15, 2016.
http://www.objnursing.uff.br/index.php/nursing/article/view/5395/pdf_1
(Accessed 19 October 2016)

[39] Turkle S: The nascent robotics culture: New complicities for companionship. AAAI Technical Series, July, 2006.

[40] Coeckelbergh M: Healthcare, capabilities, and AI assistive technology. Ethical Theory and Moral Practice, Vol. 13, pp. 181-190, 2010.
DOI: 10.1007/s10677-009-9186-2

[41] Pine A: From healing to witchcraft: On ritual speech and roboticization in the hospital. Cult Med Psychiatry, Vol. 35, pp. 262-284, 2013.
DOI: 10.1007/s11013-011-9214-2

163

Part 3

[42] Winner L: The whale and the reactor. University of Chicago, Chicago, 1986.

[43] Will robots need their own ethics?

https://philosophynow.org/issues/72/Will_Robots_Need_Their_Own_Ethics

(Accessed 20 October 2016)

[44] Almerud S, Alapack R, Fridlund B, Ekebergh M: Caught in an artificial split: a phenomenological study of being a caregiver in the technologically intense environment. Intensive and Critical Care Nursing, Vol. 24, pp.130-136, 2008.

DOI: 10.1016/j.iccn.2007.08.003

[45] Barnard A: Nursing and the primacy of technological progress. International Journal of Nursing Studies, Vol. 36, pp. 435-442, 1999.

DOI: 10.1016/S0020-7489(99)00050-4

[46] Technology to Watch in the Nursing Practice: Robotics. American Sentinel (May 31, 2016).

http://www.nursetogether.com/technology-watch-nursing-practice-robotics

(Accessed 18 October 2016)

[47] Barnard A: Alteration to will as an experience of technology and nursing. Journal of Advanced Nursing, Vol. 31, pp. 1136-1144, 2000.

DOI: 0.1111/j.1365-2648.2000.tb03460.x

[48] Barnard A: A critical review of the belief that technology is a neutral object and nurses are its master. Journal of Advanced Nursing, Vol. 26, pp. 126-131, 1997.

DOI: 0.1046/j.1365-2648.1997.1997026126.x

[49] Faltholm Y, Jansson A: Telephone advisory services-nursing between organisational and occupational professionalism. New Technology, Work and Employment, Vol. 23, pp. 17-29, 2008. DOI: 10.1111/j.1468-005X.2008.00200.x

[50] McGrath M: The challenges of caring in a technological environment: critical care nurses' experiences. Journal of Clinical Nursing, Vol. 17, pp. 1096-1104, 2008.

DOI: 10.1111/j.1365-2702.2007.02050.x.

[51] Barnard A: Radical nursing and the emergence of technique as healthcare technology. Nursing Philosophy, Vol. 17, pp. 8-18, 2016. DOI: 10.1111/nup.12103

164

Abstract

This chapter describes the Transactive Relationship Theory of Nursing (TRETON) as a middle-range theory, grounding the process of nursing as a technological and mutual engagement in nursing encounters – interrelated events between healthcare robots and human persons occurring in human healthcare environments. Theory-based nursing practice is appreciated within an ethical milieu.

Key Words: Nursing, Caring, Healthcare robots, Human persons, Technological engagements, Mutual engagements, Nursing encounters, Knowing person

Chapter XI

The Transactive Relationship Theory of Nursing (TRETON): A Model for Nursing Engagement of Healthcare Robots and Human Persons

By Tetsuya Tanioka

165

Part 3

1. Introduction

The aging population in Japan has increased and continues to increase at a phenomenal rate unequaled in any other country [1]. This phenomenon signifies that the population of older persons and in particular those with dementia is also continually increasing. It is predicted that by the year 2025, one out of every ten older adults will suffer from dementia [2]. In addition, the declining birth rate associated with the aging society has similarly contributed to this changing population demographic structure [3].

Furthermore, while the aging population is increasing, the working-age group has not caught up with the trend. This situation has expectedly become a serious social problem, leading to labor shortages, particularly within healthcare settings. This scarcity of labor is more distinctly recognized among nurses and other direct-care health caregivers. Particularly in settings demanding relationship-based nursing care, such as in older adult care institutions, there is a need for warm and compassionate human caring. This scarcity of human resources means Japan will not be able to meet this demand. Reacting to this phenomenon, Japan has made a national commitment focused on the development of healthcare robots for the older adult population (Japan Times News, 2016).

Research on robots that assist patients in physically transporting themselves [4], or that perform simple tasks like taking vital signs or delivery [5, 6] is critically needed. Reducing these types of human-dependent activities will, more importantly, allow human nurses to focus on direct human caring relationships and nursing care for these patients. Furthermore, healthcare robot research is urgently needed to focus on developing new computational algorithms for determining accurate patient emotional state classification in interactions between human and intelligent machine relations with healthcare robots during healthcare services [7].

In response to these identified needs and demands, studies have been conducted which focused on topics such as "what is a healthcare robot?" and "what nursing tasks physically performed by human nurses can be performed efficiently by

166

Chapter XI

healthcare robots?" or "what are the possibilities healthcare robots play in stereotypical human nurse behaviors?" Because nursing care is more than the completion of tasks that healthcare robots can perform, it is not appropriate to define nursing care as the performance of tasks that healthcare robots do. It is now a reality that technical capabilities possessed by healthcare robots are dramatically evolving, answering some or most of the aforementioned questions.

Moreover, some extant studies that currently inform the topic of healthcare robots' functionalities include: "Performance Requisites for Compassionate Nursing Care Robots" [8], "Empathic understanding in human-robot communication" [9, 10], "Artificiality in intelligence of human caring machines" [11], "Nursing Robot's Capability/Feasibility and Ethical Issues" [12-14], "Required Functions of the Caring Robot with Dialogue Abilities for Patients with Dementia" [15], and "Functions of a Caring Robot in Nursing" [5]. The results of these studies direct the futuristic consideration of perfecting a "real" healthcare robot that can assist with the demands of human caring in nursing, particularly among older adults and those with dementia.

As the health statuses of patients change, it will be necessary to verify the extent of the needs and demands for healthcare, and to explore whether or not robots can actually share in the fullness of nursing care, such as in situations requiring competent assessments and timely judgments or whether or not caring or the functionality of healthcare robots is a major assistance to the tasks of nursing.

Ethical and moral issues have challenged experts of nursing and engineering in Japan and in the broader global community. However, while there exists a need to address the functionalities of healthcare or caring robots, little discussion has been done for the most part on the introduction of these robots into healthcare settings. What is important to understand, however, is the apparent apathy that nursing professionals have shown towards nurses, healthcare or caring robots, and similarly, as Ito, et al. [16, 17] have found, the lack of interest from nursing experts on the existence and use of intelligent machines in healthcare settings and their lack of current information about them.

167

Part 3

2. Purpose

The purpose of this paper is to describe the Transactive Relationship Theory of Nursing (TRETON), a middle-range theory grounded in the theories of Nursing as Caring [18], and *Technological Competency as Caring in Nursing* [19]. Revealed in this theory is a practical process of relationship advanced as the transactive engagement between human persons (patients) and caring or healthcare (nurse) robots as intelligent machines. As such, the theory illustrates a unique and emerging theory-based practice of nursing.

2.1. The Transactive Relationship Theory of Nursing (TRETON)

The realization of human and intelligent machine transactions in human healthcare has been the impetus for the development of the TRETON. As the demands and needs for quality healthcare rise, particularly in environments poor in human resources and among the older adult population, the use of human-machine process requirements is intensified, and the realities and consequences of transactive relationships have become integral to assuring quality human healthcare.

"Transactive" is a term that focuses on the transactional nature of things. As an active process within the theory, it illuminates the main feature of the relationship between human-to-human and human-to-intelligent machines, which is that it is always a transaction. The term delineates as well as illuminates the relationship between caring or healthcare robots and human persons (patients). TRETON is a theoretical transactive engagement, and as such, the process of nursing is an "active" engagement between the nurse and person being nursed.

Some of the concerns, demands, and needs which have influenced the development of this theory include:

- The functionality of healthcare robots as a requirement for assisting in human caring.
- The possibility that older adults with dementia can gain well-being from dialogues and conversations with healthcare robots.

Chapter XI

• The need for theories guiding nursing practice with healthcare robots.

Accordingly, the following questions are posited:

• If healthcare robots are developed and introduced into healthcare facilities for older adults, should not the ethical issue of robotic practice engagements be prioritized and fully discussed and addressed for realizable solutions?

• What functionalities may be required of healthcare robots to engage in a compassionate, nurturing relationship within the demands of robot performance?

• Should nurses and other key healthcare personnel still provide the required healthcare tasks and practices considering human-to-human relationships, and between humans and healthcare robots?

These questions advance the TRETON as focused on the constant and "active" transactional engagement between the nurse, the healthcare robot, and patient triad.

2.2. Background

The overwhelming development of personal computers, the intranet and the Internet is transforming the work methods of nurses, doctors/physicians, and other healthcare staff members who work in hospital settings. Two of the most distinctive technologies available and used in current healthcare settings are the ordering systems and the use of electric care cards [20].

The functionalities of these technologies are irreplaceable. For example, when a patient undergoing an examination at an internal medicine clinic is given an order for a prescription, the ordering system makes it possible to send that data to each department instantly. By using electric cards, clinical data and nursing data are recorded and shared with multiple professionals.

In addition, it has become possible to select what is needed through a simple click of the gadget, thereby keeping track of the prescription as well as the information of plans for nursing stored in the database. All these are realized by using Artificial Intelligence (AI).

169

Part 3

3. Artificial intelligence and healthcare robots features

Shanahan [21] explained that "The idea that human history is approaching a 'singularity' – in that ordinary humans will someday be overtaken by artificially intelligent machines or cognitively enhanced biological intelligence, or both – has moved from the realm of science fiction to serious debate" (https://mitpress.mit.edu/books/technological-singularity). The Singularity, "a hypothetical moment in time when AI and other technologies have become so advanced that humanity undergoes a dramatic and irreversible change" (https://en.oxforddictionaries.com/definition/ singularity), is a critical influence on the development of healthcare robots and thus becomes a major concern in the appreciation of practicing nursing with these robots possessing AI capabilities.

The introduction of AI has reliably increased the speed of healthcare operations particularly in hospital settings, supporting the anticipation and realization that AI has a more expansive future. Healthcare robots would change human relationships, particularly between human persons as patients and nurses. In view of this, what is most important is that nurses actively participate in the introduction of healthcare robots into resource-poor settings, help design and test their functionality. Also important is the concern regarding the relationship between nursing judgment and the use of databases. By using nursing judgment in thirteen areas of North American Nursing Diagnosis Association (NANDA), Nursing Outcome Classification (NOC), and Nursing Intervention Classification (NIC), a description of the manner and kind of observations and care given is accounted for, so that a necessary nursing plan can be made. However, as a technological system, it is possible that technical problems will occur.

There are two common possible problems identified. Firstly, in the case that a nurse uses NANDA just as if it was a simple manual, the healthcare robot with AI capabilities will inevitably function only as an old-fashioned robot. This means that the impersonal aspect of technology is perceived to de-emphasize the need to know the patient and act as a distraction from the nurse-patient relationship. In situations

170

Chapter XI

such as these, nurses are torn between the human caring model of nursing and the robot-like attitudes perceived to be created by technology [22] or other prescriptive data bases such as NANDA, NOC, and NIC.

The other possible problem is that if a nursing plan is made automatically without any information derived from conversations/discussions between patients and nurses, knowledge about the patients will not be current, and nursing care will become mechanical – without actually knowing and understanding the patient as human person and his/her unique needs or hopes for well-being.

It is useful to take advantage of this and understand that with these databases, technological systems as nursing diagnosis are recognized as empirical ways of knowing the person. However, it is most important to note that to be functional, technological competency ought to be understood and appreciated as an expression of care in nursing. The expression of nursing between the concepts of caring and technology is advanced by Locsin [19] in the middle range theory of *Technological Competency as Caring in Nursing.*

4. Developing the Transactive Relationship Theory of Nursing (TRETON)

The Transactive Relationship Theory of Nursing acknowledges ways in which human-to-human and human-to-intelligent machine nursing encounters are expressed in nursing. It is a critical and much-needed theory from which is derived a practical process of nursing as a transactive engagement expressed as nursing transpiring between the nurse and nursed – the shared engagement between human persons (patients) and intelligent machines (healthcare robots). The engagement is an active one occurring within the nursing encounter between the nurse and nursed, co-existing in a transactive relationship (Fig. 11-1).

171

Part 3

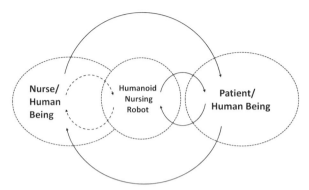

Humanoid nursing robots' ability to remember which is critical in order to share the patient's experiences; the ability to process language and maintain a conversation; and to read and illustrate emotions.

Fig. 11-1: The relationships between and among nurses, humanoid nursing robots, and patients

The nursing encounter is what Boykin and Schoenhofer [18] describes as a "nursing situation", the shared lived experience in which the caring between the nurse and nursed enhances personhood. Similarly, it is also what Locsin [23] has called the technological encounter of a co-created moment in which the nursed and nurse, through technologies of care, come to know each other more fully as caring persons. How will this process of transactive engagement guide the practice of nurses in human-healthcare robot nursing encounters?

5. Theoretical assumptions

- **Nursing is a relationship between and among human beings (human persons) and intelligent machines (healthcare robots).**

AI influences healthcare robot functionality. AI is necessary in healthcare robots. In order to express caring in nursing, healthcare robots are used to enhance the quality of nursing care by the "delegation" of healthcare tasks to

Chapter XI

the robots – not to solve the nursing care problem, nor meet the demands of task completion because of shortage of nurses or other health caregivers.

- **Nurses use technologies of care for practice.**

Nurses are adept at technologies that aid the practice of nursing. However, an understanding of and intentionality with the code of ethical practice for nurses guides the suitable use of AI in hospitals and in other healthcare arenas. Nurses must always exercise sensibility with AI-capable equipment. Transactive relationships are guided by ethical use of AI in nursing.

- **Intelligent machines possess AI that can mimic human interactions.**

Various levels of AI provide "intelligent" versions of humanoid robots capability of interactive discourse and seamless physico-mechanical movements. Today, robots abound in healthcare institutions: from guided delivery of "containers" of medications, to automated security systems, surgical instrumentations, and interactive telemachines. The AI of healthcare robots gives them the ability to engage in practical relationships, to possess high-level AI programming, and to extend interactive discourse with human persons.

- **Human-to-intelligent machine relationships are technology dependent.**

From mobility to physical capabilities, robots depend on sophisticated technologies – from enhanced robotic performance to "super-intelligent" discursive abilities.

- **Transactive relationships are guided by ethics in nursing.**

Regardless of the level of sophistication in physico-mechanical functions and intelligence, healthcare robots are expected to have a programmed response system that is guided by ethico-moral sensibilities. The possible problem that may arise in potentially contradictory situations is the dependency that robots may encounter in relationship situations, simply because it is dependent on human coded programs (Fig. 11-2).

173

Part 3

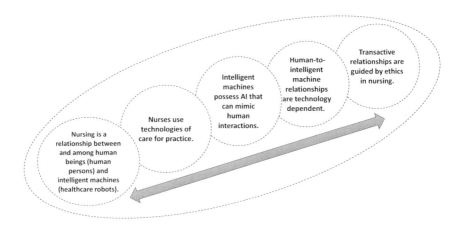

Fig. 11-2: Assumptions of the Theory of Transactive Relationships in Nursing (TRETON)

6. Evolving healthcare robots as intelligent machines

Fundamental questions exist that challenge the development of healthcare robots. These include: (1) What is healthcare and nursing? (2) Should healthcare robots be humanoids? (3) What necessary functions are required for these robots so that their performance of delegated healthcare tasks can be enhanced? (4) What level of intelligence should a healthcare robot have so that it can function effectively as a responsive "assistant" to human persons as patients? (5) Up to which levels of decision-making should healthcare robots have to be a dependable partner assisting in solving patient-care problems? (6) What ethical issues for a healthcare robot exist as it is introduced to medical institutions or hospitals? These questions warrant answers that help foster understanding of human-to-intelligent machine interrelationships.

The transaction that occurs between machine technologies and human beings originate from the perceived desire of assuring the quality of patient care now and in

Chapter XI

the future. In so doing, a guide for practicing nursing from the perspective of mechanical technologies and caring in nursing is presented as integral to ensuring the quality of patient care, with intelligent machines as primary characters within the transactive relationship.

Therefore, nurses must have a deep understanding of the code of ethical nursing practice to guide the introduction of new technologies and their usefulness in perpetuity. There are no common conceptions of ethico-moral practices within all cultures and so the ethics of care in one country may not be accepted in another country. Similarly, healthcare robots care for patients following AI-namely, instructed activities based on human-made programs because all robot-programming is accomplished by human beings. However, this may change in the future, when robot technologies and AI surpass human ingenuity.

7. Enhancing nursing and caring in healthcare robots

If healthcare robots are to be developed and introduced into hospitals and other healthcare facilities – and specifically for the older adult population – then ethical issues for practice engagements must be discussed and addressed with realizable co-created solutions. The basic function of healthcare robots is to support nurses and enhance patient healthcare. It will become necessary for healthcare robots to be equipped with the functionality to recognize and respond to the emotional expressions of persons [8]. Caring is an intentional expression of Nursing and in this case, it also carries an expectation that healthcare robots in the future will be able to assist with this. Healthcare robots may be delegated to "be with", to "listen to", to "gently touch", and assist with other caring behaviors programmed into its system.

Caring is a concept central to professional nursing practice and discipline [24]. Since the time of Florence Nightingale, the goal of nursing has remained unchanged, i.e. to provide a safe and caring environment that promotes patient health and well-being [25]. Mayeroff [26] in his book *On Caring* provided a detailed

175

Part 3

description and explanation of the encounters of caring by and being cared for. Since then nursing theorists grounded in caring have been studying the relationships between nursing and caring. Mayeroff [26] has articulated that there are basic ingredients of caring expressed between a parent who is caring for a child, a teacher who is caring for a pupil, a psychotherapist caring for a patient, or a husband caring for his wife. They all exhibit a common pattern of caring even though such caring may be uniquely expressed.

Other ingredients of caring by Mayeroff [26] include: honesty, courage, hope, knowing, patience, trust, humility, and alternating rhythms. These ingredients are useful in helping one to understand the ambiguous concept of caring, as one is called to reflect on how each of these ingredients is lived uniquely every day. This understanding of living caring, and knowing the self as caring is the basis for knowing the other as caring.

Similarly, Boykin and Schoenhofer [27] stated that the caring that is nursing must be a lived experience of caring between the nurse and the person being nursed, communicated intentionally, and with an authentic presence through an interconnectedness, a sense of oneness with self and other. They [27] declared that the knowing of nursing is embedded within the nursing situation, defined as a shared lived experience in which the caring between the nurse and nursed enhances personhood. Thoughtful reflection upon practical nursing situations provides exquisite opportunities for uncovering the knowledge and essence of caring in nursing.

Moreover, Locsin [19] explained the connection between technology and caring in nursing. Specifically, technological competency as caring in nursing is the effective use of technologies which allow nurses to understand patients more fully as whole persons and in doing so, understand patients' "calls for nursing" and respond accurately and appropriately to their hopes, dreams, and aspirations for living and growing in caring. The complementary system of "calls for nursing" and "response" builds up trusting relationships between human persons as patients and nurses.

176

Chapter XI

8. The nursing encounter: Where all nursing occurs

The occurrence of a nursing relationship exists between and among human-to-human and human-to-intelligent machines. The ***nursing encounter*** is the focal point of engagement between the nurse and nursed. Two distinctive features of this engagement are the human-to-human relationship between the human nurse and human patient, and the ***technological engagement*** between the humanoid robot - the intelligent machine – and the patient in "its" care. As technological engagements occur, the nursing encounter is illuminated as the shared experience in which the nursing encounter is explained, fostering good human caring. In order to acknowledge the value of understanding these encounters, the necessary element of "knowing" the patient is initiated.

As one of the central characters in this nursing encounter is a highly evolved intelligent machine, technological knowing [23] becomes an essential dimension in this initial stage of knowing. In appreciating the nursing encounter – the occasion in which the transactive relationship through technological knowing occurs – ***mutual engagements*** transpire. Such a relationship is much like Locsin's [28] mutual designing, an elemental dimension in the practice process of the *Technological Competency as Caring in Nursing* theory. If the healthcare robot and the human person assume the participants-in-their-care role, the patient may passively or actively participate in creating a plan of care addressing the desire towards well-being or more-being [29] or of enhanced personhood [18], i.e. living the meaning of one's own life (Fig. 11-3).

177

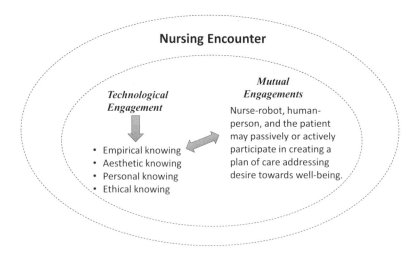

Fig. 11-3: Transactive engagement: The process of nursing

Moreover, in the healthcare setting a variety of technology is introduced; the ultimate form of providing care through the use of AI technology is considered humanoid robot activities. These activities performed by intelligent machines, expressed as tenderness or caring within the human – technology interactions become practices which are much like those activities human beings do, thereby easily appreciated as similar to human-to-human caring. This is the ultimate form of the human-to-intelligent machine transactive relationship, the rationale following the dual features of the theory-based practice in human-to-human, and human-to-intelligent machine engagements.

Today, the usefulness of healthcare robots may be about the functionalities of physical care for patients – for example those requiring change of patient clothing – and continuous monitoring of vital signs, to name a few. In order for healthcare robots to recognize humans, they have to exist in the world of the patients. In order for healthcare robots to be in the world of those receiving nursing care, consent from the patients and other healthcare staff needs to be secured. Patients have a right to decide whether or not to allow nurses and healthcare robots to collect and store their

Chapter XI

personal information and medical histories. This consent for nursing care and the acquisition of health information should be sought upon admission.

It is necessary for professional nurses and patients to fully understand the usefulness of healthcare robots and the elements of delegated care. Patient cooperation and patient safety are assured when an understanding among all participants is reached, in that the patient understands that the professional nurse has delegated certain healthcare tasks to the robots, but also that the nurse remains responsible for the tasks performed by the robot. It is also crucial to obtain permission from the patient because they need to check whether nurses are suited to care for them so that they could build a relationship of confidence. However, in the case of healthcare robots, it is critical that patients – as well as human – nurses see to it that healthcare robots are indeed trustworthy. This is an element of Delegation. The nurse delegates healthcare tasks to the delegate, which in this instance is the healthcare robot, but still retains responsibility for the care provided.

9. Concerns about healthcare robots characteristics

There are two possible problems with the introduction of healthcare robots. First, there is an ethical problem. Human nurses are licensed to provide nursing care, the license guaranteeing the nurse's competence to provide nursing care including assessments, decision-making, and the competent use of technologies. However, for the moment, there is no similar standard for healthcare robots. Nurses must consider how the quality of the robots' performance of their specific tasks are ensured. Secondly, if nurses are not included in decisions about the appropriate use of healthcare robots, then engineers or business giants will make the crucial decisions. If these issues are solved and the government bestows nursing licenses to healthcare robots, then the robots will become assistive colleagues of nurses and be able to work at hospitals.

As healthcare robots are actually "personalized" AI, their capabilities may be below the level of humans, and it is natural that we should consider them as

179

Part 3

assistants to nurses. However, today, some robots with AIs have the ability to improve themselves through activity encounters just like humans do [30]. Looking to the future, one can see the possibility that robots with AI will exceed human intelligence, i.e., when scientific advancement brings to existence robots with super AI and with high functions of learning [31]. Furthermore, what is important is the possibility of robots with AI creating their own AI.

However, it is provable that AI with the intelligence and information-processing skills of human nurses will soon be available in healthcare institutions. Is it then possible that healthcare robots will exceed nurses' capacity to provide professional care and assume their roles?

10. Performance of healthcare robots in a transactive relationship

What abilities may be required of healthcare robots to "practice" nursing as human caring within the demands of robot performance? Anthropomorphic machines are embodied mechanical entities interacting with humans [32]. The performance of these machines ought to focus on their *ability to remember*, which is critical in order to share the patient's experiences; the *ability to process language and maintain a conversation*; and the *ability to read and illustrate emotions* from facial expressions – these will all become necessary functions. Essentially, in various healthcare settings, it will be necessary to facilitate and encourage conversations centering on the relationship between "human" as well as the conversations between "human and human", and eventually among "human and healthcare robot".

The practice of nursing requires the ability of nurses to understand patients. Therefore robots should also possess this ability, so that they may be able to practice healthcare similar to humans; or better, the robots may also be required to possess high-level thinking properties/processes, such as empathy, confidence, and conscience. The five human senses will all become their requisite characteristics [33]. In order to function like human nurses, these healthcare robots must show an

180

understanding of patients based on some level of expertise and conscience, and the ability to express themselves humanely, including being empathic and kind.

Moreover, in nursing relationships, the nurses also need to grow alongside the patients. What does it mean when human nurses grow in their caring [26]? Nurses learn from the patients through encounters, and they grow in their experiences which can influence future practice. For this reason, it may be necessary to develop self-enhancing AI healthcare robots, assuming that these intelligent machines can record empirical knowledge onto their specific databases – an AI system equivalent to a human brain. In this situation, the healthcare robot can share experiences with other human nurses, healthcare robots, and other similar instances as legally sanctioned by law.

Furthermore, while Travelbee's [34] interpersonal model of nursing focuses on human-to-human relationships, it is also important to understand the specific concept of human relationships – a feature of engagement that can be an outstanding feature of a healthcare robot with a sophisticated AI.

11. Healthcare robots and knowing in nursing

Knowing a person is a central feature of human caring; and healthcare robot caring practice – if it is to be significantly valuable to nursing and human healthcare – must be able to sanction such activities as knowing persons. Nurses are required to make good use of these healthcare robots and thereby help them understand human persons (patients) more fully. Nursing does not only require technical skillfulness, which healthcare robots can excel at, but also the ability to communicate to patients with compassion, an understanding of humans getting better, and the ability to make ethical judgments accurately and appropriately. In the practice of nursing, knowing is the essential process that initiates the relationship between the nurse and nursed. While Carper [35] has described four fundamental patterns of knowing in nursing, knowing the other person continually and intentionally leads to the understanding of persons more fully as persons. All persons have aspects of self that they can change

Part 3

from moment to moment, therefore, healthcare robots have to use a process of "knowing" in order to understand the person from moment to moment.

Guided by Carper's [35] fundamental patterns of knowing in nursing, the technological engagement in the transactive relationship between human persons and intelligent machines is best expressed through patterns of knowing.

Personal knowing:

In nursing, nurses make efforts to share experiences with care participants (human persons as patients) through human connections. In doing so, nurses know and understand the other person. Personal knowing is to recognize images, fingerprints, and the individual persons. They record information regarding conversations with their patients and record these in databases such as the electronic medical/health care record. These recorded data can be shared by those authorized to access these data, and sharing these with the patients and other healthcare personnel enables them to know and understand their patients more fully as persons.

Similarly, healthcare robots have databases. Through programmed technological capabilities, they are able to collect and store data, and at appropriate times interpret these data, somewhat understanding them at the robots' level of intelligence. Healthcare robots can measure vital signs electronically and assess a patient's physical condition and emotions by recognizing facial expressions and through interactive engagements. Moreover, they can conduct recordings necessary for nursing care through sound recognition, particularly when they are paired with human nurses. In order to provide sufficient care by using scientific information such as anatomical, physiological, and pharmacological data, healthcare robots strive to analyze and interpret the whole image of care of the human person (patient) by considering their anxieties and their psychological responses to their prospective healthcare treatments. Sensory data are not lacking with healthcare robots. Their capacities continually increase exponentially.

Chapter XI

Empirical knowing:

Nurses should consider the participants' biological, psychological, sociological, cultural, medical, and spiritual conditions – including their psychological state – in order to create appropriate and accurate nursing care activities. In nursing care institutions, nursing skills mean technological expertise such as measuring blood pressure, heart rate, and body temperature, and also observing the patient's physical situation. The data collected from these processes are automatically transferred from the measuring equipment to the database. Healthcare robots can also do the same provided its programming includes certain parameters that measure certain conditions. For one, it can confirm the remaining amount of intravenous drip and instantly provide this information to nurses.

Healthcare robots can obtain the latest information regarding the patients' medical treatment, rehabilitation, and other care methods necessary in conducting appropriate and accurate nursing care. Similarly, for various illnesses, healthcare robots can gain access to databases and from the internet so that human nurses and healthcare robots can jointly judge the patient's situation. If healthcare robots gain access to the internet and provide the most appropriate information to nurses as well as patients through AI, healthcare robots can help them make a well-informed decision.

Ethical knowing:

In order to care, nurses should practice nursing within the viewpoint of what is good, right, and best for the patients. However, in addition to common sense and ethical judgment, it would be very difficult to introduce personal judgment between right or wrong into healthcare robots because there are no strict standards, even for humans. Nevertheless, this functionality can be added in rudimentary form and then enhanced exponentially given the current degree of technological sophistication.

Aesthetic knowing:

In order to communicate what the nurse knows about the patient through his or her knowing, the nurse needs to express this knowledge in ways that others can appreciate. So that nurses realize the care recipient's wishes, or help them grow as

183

Part 3

caring persons as they meander through the maze of human healthcare, they need to reflect on the caring process and consider how to provide even better, more convenient, and more responsive care.

For example, for his purpose, the nurse asks the patient's latest wish or current desire, and the patient takes time deciding his desires, hopes, dreams and aspirations. Human nurses may be able to capture these essences and the accumulated data can be stored in databases. Moreover, personal effects such as photographs, and laboratory information can be stored and made available to family members when appropriate. Information related to past experiences including those of their parents are inserted into the database as accessible information. In this sense, it is important to program into the robots such an interactive relationship. Therefore, in order to have healthcare robots function within the Transactive Relationship Model, it is necessary to develop a computerized interface communication process between healthcare robots and healthcare practitioners.

12. Concluding statements emphasizing nursing practice applications

The increasing population of older persons worldwide fosters increasing realization of the need of a theory-based practice model that can guide professional nursing practice in situations where healthcare robots engage with human persons (patients). Being critical participants in the process of human healthcare, healthcare professionals have envisioned that transactive engagements of older adults with healthcare robots may be possible in the next few decades. A theory-guided nursing practice is integral to meet the demands of this vulnerable population. Attaining good quality healthcare particularly in situations in which human beings, robots, and patients are involved may be the common healthcare practice in the very near future.

Nursing caring practices involving intelligent machines with highly sophisticated robotic functions such as interactive capabilities may be the best option for the care of the increasing older adult population. Engaging in activities

184

Chapter XI

that assure good health within the changing and evolving world of human caring is essential for human healthcare.

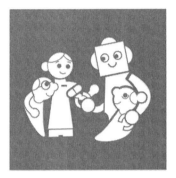

- Verbal and nonverbal communication
- Facial expression
- Eye contact
- Touching for person
- Knowing person and sharing lived experience in the nursing situation

Healthcare robots should be able to correspond according to the mood, feeling, and emotion, including expressions of suffering.

Nurses are required to make good use of Humanoid nurse robots thereby understanding patients more fully. Elderly persons can gain well-being from dialogues and conversations with Humanoid nurse robots.

Fig. 11-4: Performance of healthcare robots in transactive relationship

The AI-equipped healthcare robot will be programmed to appreciate the meanings of the nursing experience. When healthcare robots are able to express themselves through humanlike emotive behaviors, they will be able to convey empathic understanding [10] in which the benefactor will be the patient (Fig. 11-4). Therefore, within the TRETON, a nursing encounter where all nursing occurs encompasses the process of nursing as technological engagement and mutual knowing. These aspects of a transactive relationship between the healthcare robot and the person being nursed essentially prepare future nursing practitioners in a highly technological world to practice appropriate and accurate nursing activities through theory-based nursing practice.

However, contemporary healthcare and its providers and participants can have the opportunity to examine the many considerations of healthcare robots providing healthcare. For example, the occurrence of nursing encounters involving human

185

Part 3

persons and healthcare robots can advance the practice of transactive engagement, but when the human person can feel to have been healed with the help of a healthcare robot, or when a human patient can be able to equate the healthcare robot to a human person practicing nursing, will this prompt the human healthcare team to possibly accept the healthcare robot as a legitimate member? If healthcare robots can demonstrate technological competency in nursing care, what will make "them" different from the type of competency in nursing as displayed by current human nurses?

Although it may be a contemporary reality that technology – regardless of having AI – may not be able to care for human persons as human nurses can, healthcare robots are being developed to assume such activity, with this question in mind: *Are they developed by nurses or others who think they know what a nurse is and what a nurse does?* However the main question still remains: *Do nursing activities and their subsequent completion make nursing care?* If so, what does nursing practice headlined by healthcare robots mean for its ontology? If the nature of healthcare robots is their assumption of human caring practices for the promotion of human health and well-being, will this nature matter, and how different will the nursing ontology this nature engenders be from the current 21st century ontology of nursing?

Still we can ask, *Why do we need healthcare robots after all?*

References

[1] Muramatsu N, Akiyama H: Japan: Super-Aging Society Preparing for the Future. The Gerontologist, Vol. 51, No. 4, pp. 425-432, 2011. DOI: 10.1093/geront/gnr067

[2] Japanese Nursing Association: Nursing for the older people in Japan, 2013. https://www.nurse.or.jp/jna/english/pdf/info-02.pdf (Accessed 19 September 2016)

[3] Bongaarts J: Human population growth and the demographic transition. Philosophical Transactions of the Royal Society of London, Vol. 364, No. 1532, pp. 2985-2990, 2009. DOI: 10.1098/rstb.2009.0137

Chapter XI

[4]   TOYOTA: TMC Shows New Nursing and Healthcare Robots in Tokyo. http://www2.toyota.co.jp/en/news/11/11/1101.html (Accessed 8 October 2016).

[5]   Huang S, Tanioka T, Locsin RC, Parker M, Masory O: Functions of a caring robot in nursing. Proceeding of 7th International Conference on Natural Language Processing and Knowledge Engineering (NLP-KE '11), pp.425-429, 2011. DOI: 10.1109/NLPKE.2011.6138237

[6]   Hirata Y, Sugiyama Y, Kosuge K: Control architecture of delivery robot for supporting nursing staff. Proceedings of 2015 IEEE/SICE International Symposium on System Integration (SII), 2015. DOI: 10.1109/SII.2015.7404944

[7]   Swangnetr M, David B, Kaber D: Emotional State Classification in Patient–Robot Interaction Using Wavelet Analysis and Statistics-Based Feature Selection. Proceeding of 2013 IEEE Transactions on Human-Machine Systems, Vol. 43, No. 1, pp. 63-75, 2013.

[8]   Tanioka T, Yasuhara Y, Osaka K, Ito H, Kato K, Sugimoto H, Locsin RC: Performance Requisites for Compassionate Nursing Robots, With Communication Competency. Proceeding of the Seventh International Conference on Information, pp. 77-80, Taipei, Taiwan, November, 2015.

[9]   Osaka K, Tanioka T, Yasuhara Y, Locsin RC: Empathic understanding in human-robot communication: Influences on caring in nursing. GSTF Conference Proceedings on WNC 2016, pp. 233-239, 2016.

[10] Osaka K, Tsuchiya S, Ren F, Tanioka T: Analysis of Empathetic Understanding Using Relationship between Electrode and Frequency. Proceeding of ICAI 2008, pp. 116-121, Beijing, China.

[11] Yasuhara Y, Osaka K, Tanioka T, Locsin RC: Artificiality in intelligence of human caring machines: Towards its effective functioning in human patient care demands. GSTF Conference Proceedings on WNC 2016, pp. 240-245, 2016.

[12] Fuji S, Ito H, Yasuhara Y, Shihong H, Tanioka T, Locsin RC: Discussion of Nursing Robot's Capability and Ethical Issues. Information: an International Interdisciplinary Journal, Vol. 17, No. 1, pp. 349-354, 2014.

187

Part 3

[13] Tanioka T, Locsin RC: Feasibility of developing nursing care robots. Proceeding of 8th International Conference on Natural Language Processing and Knowledge Engineering (NLP-KE '12), pp. 567-570, China, 2012.

[14] Ito H, Yasuhara Y, Tanioka T, Locsin RC: Adoption of medical/welfare robots in medical environments and its ethical issues. Proceeding of 8th International Conference on Natural Language Processing and Knowledge Engineering (NLP-KE '12), pp. 560-562, China, 2012.

[15] Yasuhara Y, Tamayama C, Kikukawa K, Osaka K, Tanioka T, Watanabe N, Chiba S, Miyoshi M, Locsin RC, Ren F, Fuji S, Ogasawara H, Mifune K: Required Function of the Caring Robot with Dialogue Ability for Patients with Dementia. AIA International Advanced Informtion Institute, Vol. 4, No. 1, pp. 31-42, 2012.

[16] Ito H, Miyagawa M, Kuwamura Y, Yasuhara Y, Tanioka T, Locsin RC: Professional Nurses' Attitudes towards the introduction of Humanoid Nursing Robots (HNRs) in Health Care Settings. Journal of Nursing and Health Sciences, pp. 73-81, 2015.

[17] Ito H, Yasuhara Y, Tanioka T, Osaka K, Locsin RC: Intelligent machines and ethical dilemmas concerning fidelity in human caring activities. GSTF Conference Proceedings on WNC 2016, pp. 228-232, 2016.

[18] Boykin A, Schoenhofer S: Nursing as Caring: A Model for Transforming Practice. Sudbury, MA: Jones Bartlett, p. 13, 2001.

[19] Locsin RC: Technological Competency as Caring in nursing. Sigma Theta Tau International Press, Indianapolis, IN, USA, 2005.

[20] Oida T, Okuyama T, Finley M: A Security Gateway System for Medical Communication Networks Inter-Hospital Use of the Secure Socket Layer. Joint International Conference on Autonomic and Autonomous Systems and International Conference on Networking and Services – (icas-isns '05), p. 35, 2005. DOI: 10.1109/ICAS-ICNS.2005.9.

[21] Shanahan M: The Technological Singularity. The MIT Press Essential Knowledge series, 2015. https://mitpress.mit.edu/books/technological-singularity (Accessed 6 October 2016)

Chapter XI

[22] Radhakrishnan K: Technology and caring: Finding common ground for nursing practice. The International Journal of Technology, Knowledge and Society, Vol. 4, No. 5, pp. 27-32, 2008.

[23] Locsin RC, Purnell M: Advancing the Theory of Technological Competency as Caring in Nursing: The Universal Technological Domain. International Journal for Human Caring, Vol.19, No. 2, pp. 50-54, 2015.

[24] Smith MC, Turkell M, Wolf Z: Caring in Nursing Classics. New York: NY, Springer, 2013.

[25] Nightingale F: Notes on Nursing: What It Is and What It Is Not. In Seymer, LR. Selected Writings of Florence Nightingale, (Ed). MacMillan Book Co., New York, 1954.

[26] Mayeroff M: On Caring. The Harper Perennial, New York, NY, 1971.

[27] Boykin A, Schoenhofer S: Nursing as Caring, A Model for Transforming Practice. Jones and Bartlett Publishers, p. 25, 1993.

[28] Locsin RC: Technological Competency as Caring in Nursing: Co-creating Moments in Nursing Occurring Within the Universal Technological Domain. The Journal of Theory Construction and Testing, Vol. 20, No. 1, pp. 5-11. 2016.

[29] Paterson JG, Zderad LT: Humanistic Nursing. New York, John Wiley & Sons, 1976.

[30] Barrat J: Our Final Invention. Thomas Dunne Books, St. Martin's Griffin Press, New York, pp. 9-31, 2013.

[31] Kurzweill R: Singularity is Near. Penguin Book, New York, 2006.

[32] Locsin RC, Tanioka T, Kawanishi C: Anthropomorphic machines and the practice of nursing: knowing persons as whole in the moment, Proceedings of 2005 IEEE International Conference on Natural Language Processing and Knowledge Engineering, IEEE NLP-KE '05, 2005. DOI: 10.1109/NLPKE.2005.1598850

[33] Miwa H, Okuchi T, Takanobu H, Takanishi A: Development of a new human-like head robot WE-4. International Conference on Intelligent Robots and Systems, IEEE/RSJ, 2002. DOI: 10.1109/IRDS.2002.1041634

[34] Travelbee J: Interpersonal Aspects of Nursing. Philadelphia. F.A. Davis, 1966.

Part 3

[35] Carper B: Fundamental patterns of knowing in nursing. Advances in Nursing Science, Vol. 1, No. 1, pp.13-24, 1978.

Abstract

This chapter explains the artificiality of intelligence necessary for humanoid robots to effectively function in human patient care situations. Also explained are the kinds of effective and responsive functioning of humanoid robots to human patients' requests, and the ethical issues arising from human-robot interactions regarding health and human care in various settings.

Key Words: Artificiality of intelligence, Ethics, Humanoid robots, Autonomous robots

Chapter XII

Artificiality of Intelligence in Human Caring Robots: Ethical Issues for Nursing

By Hirokazu Ito, Yuko Yasuhara, Kyoko Osaka, Tetsuya Tanioka, Rozzano C. Locsin

Part 3

1. Introducing for nursing robot to medical environment

1.1. Current state of robot engagements in Japan

Japan is facing a super-aging society where the elderly population, those older than 65 years old, accounts for more than 25% of the total population. This percentage is expected to increase to 40% by 2055 [1]. The development and introduction of robots in Japanese industry, particularly in healthcare, is accelerating rapidly. Currently, there are varieties of robots in healthcare institutions while robot industries are producing many more. For example, there are now robots which can assist in surgery – nearly 200 units are used with great interest because of the precision and efficiency that these robots can guarantee [2, 3]. Additionally, in 2016 the Japan Agency for Medical Research and Development (AMED) has pursued the implementation of the large-scale study (19 types, 1000 robots) of robots to analyze the effect of introducing communication robots in nursing [4].

1.2. Challenges in the use of humanoid robots

Can humanoid nursing robots (HNRs) touch the patient in their performance of nursing care? Nurses and other healthcare providers are practicing nursing in accordance with the Medical Care Law in Japan. This law allows nurses to care for patients guided by the Act on Public Health Nurses, Midwives and Nurses. Similarly, in Japan, it is considered that the user (healthcare provider) and manufacturers of humanoid robots have the utmost responsibility towards assuring their safe and precise performance. If humanoid robots cause injuries to patients, the parties involved – such as the robot seller, medical staff, and hospital organizations – hold the legal responsibility. However, there is a limit in the current statutes of Japan's Medical and Welfare Law as regards the unintentional injuries caused by robots.

In 2014, the International Organization for Standardization (ISO) issued ISO 13482, an international standard on the safety of personal care robots [5-7]. ISO 13482:2014 specifies requirements and guidelines for the inherently safe design, protective measures, and information for use of personal care robots. Currently,

192

Chapter XII

there are three types of personal care robots: the mobile servant robot; the physical assistant robot; and the person carrier robot. These robots typically perform tasks to improve the quality of life of their intended users, irrespective of age or capability. ISO 13482:2014 describes hazards associated with the use of these robots, and provides requirements to eliminate, or reduce, the concomitant risks to an acceptable level. ISO 13482:2014 covers human-robot physical contact applications.

1.3. Hazards of using humanoid robots

ISO 13482:2014 presents significant hazards in the use of personal care robots and describes how to deal with them for each (humanoid) robot type. ISO 13482:2014 covers robotic devices used in personal care applications which are treated as activities performed by personal care robots. ISO 13482:2014 is limited to earthbound robots.

However, ISO 13482:2014 does not apply to robots travelling faster than 20 km/h such as robot toys, or water-borne and flying robots. Industrial robots are covered in ISO 10218, including robots used as medical devices, or military or public force application robots. The scope of ISO 13482:2014 is limited primarily to human care-related hazards but, where appropriate, it also includes domestic animals or household property (defined as safety-related objects), when the personal care robot is properly installed and maintained and used for its intended purpose or under conditions which can reasonably be foreseen.

ISO 13482:2014 is not applicable to robots manufactured prior to its publication date. This international standard is focused on the safety of personal care robots. However, it is a new field of ISO and a pertinent issue is that there is no accumulation of risk assessment viewpoints. It is necessary that national societies and the world community, and those responsible for introducing these robots to healthcare settings [8], be cognizant of the risks and hazards of using these types of intelligent machines. Legal improvements in medical equipment, healthcare robots, and in the social aspects of patient and healthcare personnel are necessary for the clinical use of rapidly advancing technology.

193

Part 3

The difference between human nurses and nurse robots should be addressed when introducing healthcare robots in the nursing care environment. This leads to the understanding of the true value of human nurses' caring in realizing "What is a nurse robot or a healthcare robot?" At present, with the accelerated development of human nurse robots, it is necessary that nurses discuss with engineers, legal professionals, politicians, patients, and hospital officials the kinds of robots and the manners of robotic capabilities that would be most desirable for introduction in the current healthcare environment.

2. Robots and human beings

2.1. Humanoid robots and ethics

Ethical views regarding humanoid robots in medical practice have changed over time due to new genetic information, to dramatic improvements in the mechanical and computer engineering fields, and on various cultural phenomena influencing attitudes of people towards humanoid robots. Ethical concerns were a consistent issue in the field of robotics and engineering. According to Noakes, et al. (2009), robot technology in the mechanical engineering field was rapidly introduced in the healthcare environment [9]; and findings in the study of Chen, et al. (2011) declared that robots will be able to have functions that can make it possible for them to communicate with humans [10].

Robots today mimic the sensitivity of human skin. The robots are now mounted with pressure sensors so that they can safely have physical contact with patients [11, 12]. Furthermore, assistance robot systems were developed and equipped with a self-traveling sensor – a welcome contraption that assists in nursing by transferring patients with precision, preventing injury. Robots are now able to safely transfer patients from bed to wheelchair and vice versa, and more securely in fact than human nurses can [13, 14].

These enhancements have given highly programmed robots advanced computing and natural language processing capabilities to respond to human directions as accurately as possible. These robots need to have a database which will exceed the storage capacity of human beings in the future. In order to create such robots, their computer programs should be developed to include appropriate computational decisions particularly in clinical settings.

2.2. Differences between human and intelligent machines

A robot by any other name is still a robot.

Unfortunately, this may not be true. Clearly, differences in humanoid robots should be discussed when introducing robots in healthcare settings. In addition, differences between humanoid robots and human nurses also require discussion. For instance, although human nurses can realize their own selves from an ontologically regarded environment, the cognitive functioning that allows this understanding is still considered premature or absent in today's intelligent humanoid robots. This means that human nurses can sense the atmosphere from surrounding environment but humanoid robots may not be able to do so. It is understood that such intelligent robots are not yet able to distinctively discriminate environmental matters such as safety, because of their limited artificial intelligence or its limited database capacity.

The discussion about differences between human and intelligent machines is most meaningful in nursing. Nurses as patient-rights advocates have continued the caring relationship between the nurses and the nursed in a medical world shaped by technology. They decide on a nursing situation appropriately and their responses regarding caring for their patients are based on sound and critical judgments, thereby building an expansive and mutual trust relationship with patients.

The use of robots and other technologies in healthcare settings bring new ethical concerns in nursing. Influenced by the development of advanced technologies, the ethical view within healthcare continues to change with the times. Therefore, a discussion based on ethical issues about the introduction of humanoid robots from the viewpoint of nurses' ethics and of society is critical and should be mandated.

195

Part 3

3. Research on contemporary ethical dilemmas of nurses and engineers concerning humanoid nursing robots development and utilization

One study (Ito, 2016) [15] sought to clarify these ethical dilemmas regarding HNRs. In this study, the functions of HNRs were explained to the participants this way: "HNRs are required to have the ability to understand patients such as their emotional behaviors and provide human caring activities as human nurses do, or assist with nursing work, not only to make up for lost nurse functions of health systems (including workforce). With abilities such as these, the possibility of healthcare provided by nurse robots will improve the overall quality of human nursing care." The participants were professional nurses and engineers who participated in international conferences in Japan, Thailand, China, the Philippines, and Taiwan. Out of a total of 600 questionnaire copies distributed, 414 were returned (there was a 69.0% response rate). Valid responses were only 386 questionnaires because some returned questionnaires had incomplete data, and/or there were errors in the data provided, such as the demographic data. The demographic data were analyzed using the remaining valid questionnaires (Tab. 12-1).

Tab. 12-1: Demographic data

		N= 386
	Nurses'	Engineers'
The number of participants	215(55.7%)	171(44.3%)
Age (Mean± SD)	36.04±14.43	26.82±12.30
Min	18	19
Max	77	65

SD: Standard Deviation, Min: Minimum, Max: Maximum

Chapter XII

84% of nurses and 67% of engineers were interested in HNRs. Nurses showed significantly higher interest than engineers (χ^2 = 15.07, p < 0.001). Of the participants who responded, 172 nurses (80.4%) and 107 engineers (62.6%) know that "HNRs will be introduced into the healthcare environment". Furthermore, nurses also showed significantly higher interest on the question of HNRs than engineers (χ^2 = 15.10, p < 0.001). However, on the question of "If you were a patient, would you accept nursing care by an HNR?" 132 nurses (61.4%) answered that they will not accept HNRs, while 100 engineers (58.5%) answered in the affirmative. The number of nurses who will not accept care by HNRs were significantly higher than engineers (χ^2 = 15.09, p < 0.001) (Tab. 12-2-a, b and c).

Tab. 12-2-a, b, and c: Relationship of interest and acceptance for HNRs

a. Are you interested in HNR?

		Yes			No				
		n	%	Adjusted Residual	n	%	Adjusted Residual	χ^2 value	p value
Nurses'	(n=214)	179	83.6	3.9	35	16.4	-3.9	15.07	<0.001
Engineers'	(n=171)	114	66.7	-3.9	57	33.3	3.9		

Pearson's χ^2 Test

b. Did you know that Robots will be introduced into the medical environment?

		Yes			No				
		n	%	Adjusted Residual	n	%	Adjusted Residual	χ^2 value	p value
Nurses'	(n=214)	172	80.4	3.9	42	19.6	-3.9	15.10	<0.001
Engineers'	(n=171)	107	62.6	-3.9	64	37.4	3.9		

Pearson's χ^2 Test

c. If you were a patient, would you accept nursing care by a HNR?

		Yes			No				
		n	%	Adjusted Residual	n	%	Adjusted Residual	χ^2 value	p value
Nurses'	(n=215)	83	38.6	-3.9	132	61.4	3.9	15.09	<0.001
Engineers'	(n=171)	100	58.5	3.9	71	41.5	-3.9		

Pearson's χ^2 Test

Part 3

Nurses (3.06 ± 1.15) had a significantly higher score than engineers (2.55 ± 1.11) regarding the statement that "HNRs should not provide care for patients" ($t = 4.36$, $p < 0.001$). Also, nurses (2.67 ± 1.27) had a significantly lower score than engineers (2.99 ± 1.05) on the topic "HNRs should provide care autonomously" ($t = -2.66$, $p < 0.05$). Nevertheless, nurses (4.01 ± 1.16) had a significantly higher score than engineers (3.56 ± 1.18) on the topic "Engineers should take responsibility if a problem occurs in patient care by an HNR" ($t = 3.79$, $p < 0.001$). It was found that nurses (4.53 ± 0.83) had a significantly higher score than engineers (3.96 ± 0.98) regarding the statement "Hospitals should take responsibility if a problem occurs in patient care by an HNR" ($t = 6.09$, $p < 0.001$). Furthermore, nurses (4.05 ± 1.17) had a significantly higher score than engineers (3.43 ± 1.15) regarding the statement "Doctors should take responsibility if a problem occurs in patient care by HNR" ($t = 5.24$, $p < 0.001$). On the topic "nurses should take responsibility if a problem occurs in patient care by HNR" ($t = 6.17$, $p < 0.001$), nurses (3.87 ± 1.28) had a significantly higher score than engineers (3.09 ± 1.18). Other highly significant results include: Nurses (4.00 ± 1.16) having a higher score than engineers (3.77 ± 0.98) on the proposition that "HNRs should provide nursing care according to the instructions of the nurse" ($t = 2.06$, $p < 0.05$). Nurses (4.24 ± 1.07) scored higher than engineers (3.65 ± 1.10) on the statement that "Ethical nursing care programs for HNRs and the safety of the patient should be assured by the nurses" ($t = 5.34$, $p < 0.001$). Nurses (4.15 ± 1.13) had a higher score than engineers (3.87 ± 1.04) regarding the statement that "Ethical nursing care programs for HNRs and the safety of the patient should be assured by the medical doctor ($t = 2.53$, $p < 0.05$)".

However, there were no significant differences in the following topics: "HNRs should provide care according to orders from human nurses"; "HNRs should provide care that is set in advance at the hospital"; "HNRs should provide minimally invasive care"; "HNRs should provide the same care as human nurses"; and "Ethical nursing care programs for HNRs and the safety of the patient should be assured by the nurse and the engineer" (Tab. 12-3).

Chapter XII

Tab. 12-3: Comparison of the difference between the average value of nurses and engineers

N=386

	Nurses' (Mean±SD)			Engineers' (Mean±SD)			t-value	p-value
1) HNRs should not provide care for patients.	3.06	±	1.15	2.55	±	1.11	4.36	***
2) HNRs should provide care autonomously.	2.67	±	1.27	2.99	±	1.05	-2.66	*
3) HNRs should provide care according to orders from human nurses.	3.89	±	1.18	3.84	±	0.92	0.43	n.s.
4) HNRs should provide care that is set in advance at the hospital.	3.49	±	1.18	3.65	±	0.97	-1.53	n.s.
5) HNRs should provide minimally invasive care.	3.56	±	1.28	3.68	±	1.02	-0.99	n.s.
6) Engineers should take responsibility if a problem occurs in patient care by a HNR.	4.01	±	1.16	3.56	±	1.18	3.79	***
7) Hospitals should take responsibility if a problem occurs in patient care by a HNR.	4.53	±	0.83	3.96	±	0.98	6.09	***
8) Doctors should take responsibility if a problem occurs in patient care by HNR.	4.05	±	1.17	3.43	±	1.15	5.24	***
9) Nurses should take responsibility if a problem occurs in patient care by HNR.	3.87	±	1.28	3.09	±	1.18	6.17	***
10) HNRs should provide the same care as human nurses.	2.96	±	1.48	3.03	±	1.24	-0.48	n.s.
11) HNRs should provide nursing care according to the instructions of the nurse.	4.00	±	1.16	3.77	±	0.98	2.06	*
12) Ethical nursing care programs for HNRs and the safety of the patient should be assured by the engineer.	4.06	±	1.22	3.86	±	1.01	1.77	n.s.
13) Ethical nursing care programs for HNRs and the safety of the patient should be assured by the nurse.	4.24	±	1.07	3.65	±	1.10	5.34	***
14) Ethical nursing care programs for HNRs and the safety of the patient should be assured by the medical doctor.	4.15	±	1.13	3.87	±	1.04	2.53	*

Student t-test and Welch test   * p<0.05, *** p<0.001 n.s.: not significant   SD= Standard Deviation
It was evaluated in by questionnaire (5) I strongly think so, (4) I think so, (3) I cannot tell for sure, (2) I don't think so, and (1) I don't think so at all.

Both the nurses and engineers were interested in HNRs. Nurses were more likely to think that HNRs will be introduced in the hospital in the future. However, concerning "whether to accept care" from HNRs, it was the nurse who replied "I will not accept care by HNRs" and not the engineer. Furthermore, many nurses responded that "HNR should not care for patients" compared to engineers.

The nurse understands the complexity of the nursing work he/she is doing. Also, nurses know that it is difficult to care for patients at the current level of HNRs' function of knowing, based on nurses' real clinical experiences. Therefore, it was suggested that nurses answered "I do not accept care from HNR". This complexity presents itself especially in older people, for they have rich life experiences, which is terribly difficult to fully empathize with, even for competent human nurses.

199

Part 3

The nurses responded that "Engineering robot developers, medical doctors, nurses, and hospitals should take responsibility for care by HNR" and not the engineers. The result was considered to be a manifestation of the nurses' responsibility in providing care to patients. The relevant clause under the heading Nurses and Practice in The International Council of Nurses (ICN) code of ethics for nurses of The ICN is as follows: "The nurse, in providing care, ensures that use of technology and scientific advances are compatible with the safety, dignity and rights of people".

It is essential to protect patients considering the influences of technological advances in patient care areas. In the background of such ethical thinking, it was suggested that nurses are guided by professional ethics.

4. Ethical issues related to Artificial Intelligence (AI)

4.1. Utilization of robots and problems with Artificial Intelligence (AI)

Ethical problems in introducing HNRs became a primary concern when a robot was involved in the sniper killings of policemen in the Dallas, USA. This robot was remote-controlled at the time of the killing, for this robot was designed and developed for disaster-relief, and works by remote control.

Considering the issue of utilization and the ethical issues of robots working in social situations, Peter Singer, a senior fellow at the nonpartisan think tank "New America" and a leading expert on 21st century security issues [16], said that many domestic police forces now have two types of robots of different sizes and shapes in their arsenal: those used for surveillance, and those used for bomb disposal. Surveillance robots are equipped, as would be expected, with cameras, while bomb disposal robots generally have a sophisticated arm that can be operated remotely by something akin to a joystick. Importantly, these robots are not designed or intended to be used as weapons to kill. However, the robot was manufactured for bomb disposal and then was used by police officers to kill a criminal. The question remains, "Is it reasonable to say that this robot was used in a way different from its

200

original use?", "What is the ethical issue in this usage?" It was the judgment call made by human law enforcement personnel that allowed the use of the police disaster-relief robots to kill a human being.

In the future, however, AI is needed to realize the ability of the humanoid robot to make its own decision, and in fact AI is critical in dispensing this "ability" and definitely making this "intelligence" indispensable. Therefore, as humanoid robots equipped with AI attain a different level of sophistication and a different level of appreciation particularly on its capacity and ability to make "intelligent" decisions, ethical dilemmas may become obsolete or be changed, for ethical laws can or may change with the times.

In 2014, Barrat has described in detail the development of AI [17], noting that fifty-six countries have been or are developing battlefield robots. AI is one of the robot features influencing ethical issues related to the introduction of robots. Scientists are now investigating AI from various specialized angles. Today, some of these features mean that AIs are used in computers, appliances, smart phones, and cars. Recent opinion polls show that computer scientists and professionals in AI-related fields such as engineering, robotics, and neuroscience are more conservative than others. They think there is a better than 10% chance that artificial general intelligence (AGI) will be created before 2028, a better than 50% chance by 2050, and a 90% chance before the end of this century.

"Singularity" has become a very popular word, even though it has several definitions that are often used interchangeably. Ray Kurzweil (2005) defines the Singularity as representing a profound and disruptive transformation in human capability [18, 19]. The non-biological intelligence created in the year 2045 will be one billion times more powerful than all human intelligence today (beginning around the year 2045). AI could drive mankind into extinction, and explaining how that catastrophic outcome may not just be possible, but likely, points out the prospect that amoral machines may dominate the intelligence realm – if we do not begin preparing very carefully now.

Part 3

4.2. HNRs and caring in nursing

HNRs equipped with AI, even if initially useful, can create a concern about whether the "friendliness" and "ethical judgment" it maintains as an intelligent machine can impact a variety of human experiences. Based on Boykin and Schoenhofer's [20] theoretical views, this concern may become relevant by asking these questions: "What about an unrepentant child rapist or a person responsible for genocide – can we say that these persons are caring, and if not, can we nurse them? Does the nurse have to like the person being nursed? Does the nurse seek enhancement of personhood in the nursing situation? If so, might the goals of the nurse be imposed on the one nursed?" When emotions expressed between HNRs (assuming HNRs possessing "super AI" have been introduced to clinical settings) are expressed in the same manner as human beings do, how can human beings create human being-HNR relationships? Transactive relationships (Tanioka, 2017) [21] among nurses, patients, healthcare personnel, and HNRs may lead to hurt feelings. Then what?

Some ethical dilemmas regarding robot use in healthcare include: HNRs possessing "super AI" may express emotions such as sadness or happiness the same way human beings do. If HNRs with human relations become technologically useless, can humans discard them? If the HNR breaks down, should human beings perform a "funeral ceremony" just like what is done with a loved one? What if the patient is upset by the actions of HNR – can the patient beat up the HNR or quarrel with it? What if the HNR is "angry", like a human being, about the patient's actions, can the HNR present a bad-tempered expression to the patient?

Various problems may be encountered in the future. However, one radical question regarding HNRs that is critical even today is, "Are HNRs the slaves of humans or are they colleagues in healthcare?"

Chapter XII

5. Conclusion

In the future, nurses may be able to accept the services of HNRs given the sophistication and uncanny realities of HNRs as partners in human nursing care. It is wise for nurses to consider accepting the services of HNRs, provided nurses are given the greater role of influencing and regulating the activities of the HNRs. Engineers and roboticists must find nurses' concerns critical to the design, development, and utilization of HNRs. Human nurses must understand fully the activities that these intelligent machines can and cannot do, and essentially accept characteristic skills and functionalities that these robots may be able to perform with more efficiency and proficiency. This way they would be able to work harmoniously. The introduction of HNRs always has the end user benefit or suffer from it, particularly from the ethico-moral dilemmas that may arise. Truly, a future consideration is the seriousness of merging developmental technologies and application utilities as the ultimate universal partnering of HNRs and human persons in human healthcare practice. What we should consider in the future is to develop HNRs to enhance the quality of people's health. In order to make HNRs the ultimate partner in human caring, human nurses must be engaged in the design and development of an HNRs' Artificial Brain.

Will HNRs be the answer to the current problematic maintenance of high quality human care? More importantly, is the specification of morally inspired robots the alternative or the mainstream healthcare practitioner of the future? The introduction of autonomous robots, humanoid robots, humanoid nurse robots, and other intelligent machines to the healthcare environment is a critically important issue, one that is integral to human health and human care. Nurses and healthcare providers should consider this phenomenon very seriously, for ultimately, the care receivers (the patients) critically determine the pros and the cons of the artificial brain of an HNR. The artificiality in human intelligence of human caring robots and the ethical issues for nursing require moral vigilance for both the practitioner of nursing and the developers of robots for human care.

203

Part 3

References

[1] Long-Term Care, Health and Welfare Services for the Elderly Ministry of Health, Lavour and Welfare (2015) Elderly Person Care of 2015 – For Establishment of the Care to Support the Dignity of the Elderly Person. (In Japanese)
http://www.mhlw.go.jp/topics/kaigo/kentou/15kourei/3a.html
(Accessed January 2016)

[2] Intuitive Surgical HP. http://www.intuitivesurgical.com/jp/aboutdavinci.html
(Accessed January 2016)

[3] Hashimoto K, Hattori K, Otani T, Lim HO, Takanishi A: Foot Placement Modification for a Biped Humanoid Robot with Narrow Feet. The Scientific World Journal, Vol. 2014, p. 9, 2014.

[4] Japan Agency for Medical Research and Development (AMED) HP.
http://www.amed.go.jp/news/release_20160518.html
(Accessed October 2016) (In Japanese)

[5] International Organization for Standardization (ISO) HP.
http://www.iso.org/iso/catalogue_detail?csnumber=53820
(Accessed November 2016)

[6] Japan Quality Assurance Organization (JQA) HP. https://www.jqa.jp/english/
(Accessed November 2016)

[7] Ministry of Economy, Trade and Industry, Japan: Japanese Service Robots were Certified under Global Safety Standard ISO13482 for the First Time in the World.
http://www.meti.go.jp/english/press/2014/0217_03.html
(Accessed November 2016)

[8] Ashrafian H: Artificial Intelligence and Robot Responsibilities: Innovating Beyond Rights, Sci Eng Ethics, 21:317–326, 2015. DOI 10.1007/s11948-014-9541-0

[9] Noakes WM, Lind FR, Jansen FJ, Love JL, Pin GF, Richardson SB: Development of a remote trauma care assist robot. Intelligent Robots and Systems. Proceedings of The 2009 IEEE/RSJ International Conference on Intelligent Robots and Systems, pp. 2580-2585, 2009.

Chapter XII

[10] Chen TL, King C, Kemp CC, Thomaz AL: Touched by a robot: An investigation of subjective responses to robot-initiated touch. Human-Robot Interaction: Proceedings of 6th ACM/IEEE International Conference, pp. 457- 464, 2011.

[11] Mukai T, Hirano S, Nakashima H, Kato Y, Sakaida Y, Guo S, Hosoe S: Development of a nursing-care assistant robot (RIBA) that can lift a human in its arms. Intelligent Robots and Systems (IROS), Proceedings of The IEEE/RSJ 2010 International Conference on Intelligent Robots and Systems, pp. 5996-6001, 2010.

[12] Kajikawa S: Development of robot hand aiming at nursing care services to humans. Robotics and Automation, Proceedings of international conference on Robotics and Automation, pp.3663-3669, 2009.

[13] Yukawa T, Nakata N, Obinata G, Makino T: Assistance system for bedridden patients to reduce the burden of nursing care. System Integration, Proceedings of IEEE/SICE International Symposium on System Integration, pp.132-139, 2010.

[14] Mukai T, Hirano S, Yoshida M, Nakashima H, Guo S, Hayakawa Y: Whole-body contact manipulation using tactile information for the nursing-care assistant robot RIBA. Intelligent Robots and Systems, Proceedings of The IEEE/RSJ 2011 International Conference on Intelligent Robots and Systems, pp. 2445–2451, 2011.

[15] Ito H, Yasuhara Y, Tanioka T, Osaka K, Locsin RC: Intelligent machines and ethical dilemmas concerning fidelity in human caring activities. Proceedings of GSTF CONFERENCE PROCEEDINGS ON WNC 2016, pp. 228-232, 2016.

[16] Time HP. http://time.com/4398196/dallas-shooting-bomb-robot/ (Accessed October 2016)

[17] James B: Our Final Invention: Artificial Intelligence and the End of the Human Era, Thomas Dunne Books, New York, pp. 16-28, 2013.

[18] The Kurzweil Accelerating Intelligence HP. http://www.kurzweilai.net/singularity-q-a (Accessed November 2016)

[19] Kurzweil R: The Singularity Is Near: When Humans Transcend Biology. Viking Books, New York, 2005.

[20] Boykin A, Schoenhofer SO: Caring: A Model for Transforming Practice. Jones & Bartlett Learning, Burlington, pp. 18-19, 2001.

205

Part 3

[21] Tanioka T: The Development of the Transactive Relationship Theory of Nursing (TRETON): A Nursing Engagement Model for persons and Robots and Humanoid Nursing Robots. Int J Nurs Clin Pract, Vol. 4, IJNCP-223, 2017.
DOI: 10.15344/2394-4978/2017/223

Abstract
This chapter describes and explains the association between humanoid robots and artificial intelligence, as well as the influence of caring in nursing and practice technologies.

Key Words: Nursing, Technologies, Caring, Humanoid robots, Artificial intelligence, Universal technological domain, Technological encounter

Chapter XIII

The Relationship among Nursing, Technologies, Caring, Humanoid Robots, and Artificial Intelligence

By Rozzano C. Locsin

Part 3

1. Introduction

The concern about robots in healthcare "practice", particularly humanoid robots, stems from the issues of artificiality in robot physiognomy (physical appearance and characteristics), their appreciation by human persons concerning its functionalities, and the imagery of intelligent machines as a menace to humanity. Theories pertinent to artificial intelligence (AI) and Robots abound, such as Isaac Asimov's Three Laws of Robots (1970 / 2012) [1], Masahiro Mori's Uncanny Valley (1971) [2], Ray Kurzweil's Singularity (2005) [3], and the ultimate AI standpoint as used in Alan Turing's test (1951) about human-computer interface [4]. Moreover, these theoretical underpinnings frequently made real in science fiction (SF) literature and films do support the anxiety, fear, and apprehension of robot dominance. Particularly, the dominance of intelligent humanoid robots with ASI (artificial superintelligence) – as Barrat (2013) [5] has appropriately declared – seems to conquer the imagination of human beings. Nevertheless, while these aspects of robots focus on the intelligent nature of machines and their utility in human society, their functionality in human healthcare particularly within the practice of nursing may assuage the fear of the horrific scenarios involving nurse robots as healthcare partners. These concerns deserve a critical deliberation regarding the philosophical and theoretical foundations of the ontological and epistemological characteristics of humanoid nurse robots (HNRs). Ito, et al. (2015) [6] have gathered nurses' attitudes in practicing and have also studied justifying their "role" based on the functionality and value of intelligent machines performing what may seem to be "nursing" in today's world.

2. Nursing practice and caring in nursing

What is nursing, and what is nursing practice? In common parlance, centered on the image of nurses and their practice, nursing is doing, i.e. performing tasks. Therefore, in view of this, the nature of nursing practice is the precise identification

208

Chapter XIII

and implementation of actions performed by the nurse, for the purpose of rehabilitating or fixing the person, thereby making the person whole again. It is this public image of the nurse particularly in hospital settings that provides a semblance of its ontological imagery; a nurse is a woman in a white uniform, often wearing a white starched cap, and dutifully performing precise activities for and sometimes with the patients. Activities such as these can include bathing, feeding, taking vital signs, making beds, assisting physicians, etc. It may seem inconceivable that this so-called "excellent nursing" practice is the outcome of four years of rigorous education involving knowing human anatomy, physiology, biochemistry, cellular physiology, pharmaco-therapeutics, etc., and the competency of practice in human engagement involving physico-physiological and interactive relations with and among other persons as patients.

Nevertheless, the study of nursing includes human caring phenomena such as responses to health-illness, caring-healing, and all the variations of being human. Nursing serves as the moral and scientific covenant that nurses have to offer as a service to humankind and society (Watson, 2012) [7]. An expanding and diverse epistemology allows not only for empirics but for the advancement of aesthetics, ethics, and personal knowing of persons as whole and complete in the moment. Nursing as a human caring science with its own ontological worldview, founded on the science of nursing, is illuminated in caring as its raison d'etre.

The science of caring is focused on the appreciation of human beings as caring persons. Mayeroff (1977) [8] has recognized and described eight ingredients that comprise "caring": namely, knowing, alternating rhythms, trust, hope, courage, honesty, patience, and humility. Likewise, Roach (1987) [9] has determined six attributes of caring: namely, compassion, competence, commitment, conscience, confidence, and comportment. Each of these attributes characterize the caring person. Guided by Boykin and Schoenhofer's (2001) [10] theory of Nursing As Caring grounding it as a transformational practice, nursing has been described as the shared lived experience of the caring between the nurse and the person being nursed.

209

Part 3

3. Consequences of nursing practice and intelligent machines

If the science of nursing is about rationalizing the actions of nurses towards the completion of tasks to fix the person or make him be whole again, it is highly likely that humanoid nurse robots will become a mainstream physical presence in environments where nursing practice is focused on fixing persons or making them be whole again, e.g. in settings like the hospital, or even in human domiciles where the expected provision of "healthcare activities" is the mainstay of home nursing practice.

However, such an expectation would mean that humanoid nurse robots will simply be technological marvels with programmed technologies comprising artificial general intelligence (AGI) [5] that can and will assist human nurses (Locsin, 2016) [11] in its "supposed" practice of nursing.

Nursing practice is more than simply performing nursing activities as "doing for" and "doing with" persons as outstanding features of human engagements. Contemporary definitions of nursing also include human engagements in supporting, affirming, and celebrating the humanness of persons (Boykin and Schoenhofer, 2001) [10], where nursing as a practice – rather than an art and a science (Bishop and Scudder, 1997) [12] – is understood and appreciated as shared experiences between nurses and the persons being nursed. In the future, it may be that the ontology and epistemology of nursing will be more than these contemporary activities.

If nursing practice remains instinctively a "doing for and doing with" patients, the practitioners of nursing may and can be replaced by autonomous technologies (humanoid nurse robots) which will be equipped with more sophisticated and programmed high-precision functions that can effectively and competently perform the tasks (Locsin, 2005) [13]. Furthermore, it is necessary that nursing and its practice be redefined, i.e. from a predictable service in which persons are understood as complete, whole, and knowable through their parts while guided by a prescribed

210

process of actions, towards a futuristic nursing practice for persons understood as whole, complete, and unpredictable.

The adaptability of nursing practice underscores the establishment of nursing as a discipline of knowledge and a practice profession. In this practice, there is no predetermined plan of care, because having one will only make human beings seem reducible to parts, and therefore predictable. Perspectives such as these only perpetuate the perception that nursing practice is the prescription of nursing actions to complete human beings, affirming the traditional understanding that it is indeed merely the completion of healthcare tasks, and that nurses' skills and techniques define its practice. Task completion follows the prescriptive process of traditional or conventional nursing, and excellent nurses were often evaluated on how well they exercised decision-making, judgment, and how skillfully they delivered technological nursing actions.

4. Knowing persons as caring in nursing: A dynamic process of nursing

Nursing is the shared engagement between the nurse and the person being nursed. Nursing care practice sustains, maintains, supports, and celebrates human health and well-being. Nursing care practices focus on activities that human nurses and autonomous nurse robots may engage with, in order to serve humankind. However, today, activities of healthcare have taken newer forms, centered on the ideals of functionalities, predictability, and the naturalness of human beings, thereby facilitating a greater appreciation of machine technologies for human caring (Locsin, 2017) [14].

Functionalities direct the actions and interactions between human persons while predictableness heightens the way human persons provide opportunities of care for appropriate and accurate human care. While demands such as this are vital to human health and well-being, the evolution of nursing practice from traditional and conservative practices to the technological revolution that has transformed

211

Part 3

healthcare into being a dependent entity trigger successful conditions and situations that forge the very naturalness of the one who cares and the one who receives care. The future of human nurse robots seems assured, given the rise of autonomous robots endowed with technological capabilities that can serve the nursing care practice well.

Knowing persons as a practice process of nursing is revealed in the knowledgeable demonstration of intentional, deliberate, and authentic encounters between persons in technologically demanding nursing practice settings, particularly those in environments requiring specialized and significant technological nursing expertise. These processes may occur together, and not necessarily as sequential events informing each occurrence as aspects of a whole.

Therefore, how does nursing occur? Nursing occurs as a caring relationship. Precision and prediction are not features of nursing, but rather the appreciation of each person as caring persons. Boykin and Schoenhofer (2001) [10] describe this shared lived experience as the "caring between" the nurse and person being nursed. Locsin (2009) [15] calls this the co-created moment of togetherness. The dynamic nursing process serves to guide the practice of nursing occurring as *technological knowing, mutual designing, and participative engaging* within the Universal Technological Domain (UTD) (Fig. 13-1).

212

Chapter XIII

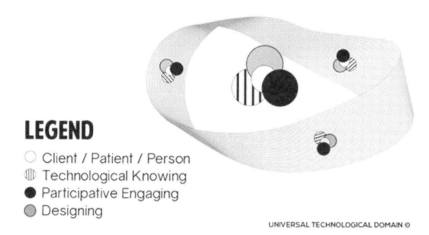

LEGEND
○ Client / Patient / Person
◐ Technological Knowing
● Participative Engaging
◎ Designing

UNIVERSAL TECHNOLOGICAL DOMAIN ©

Fig. 13-1: Illustration of the universal technological domain

Furthermore, true nursing is something that is modified based on the human interaction between the nurse and person being nursed (Tanioka, 2017) [16]. In a continuously changing society, the future of nursing is technological knowing expressed within nursing engagements derived from patient situations and their familial contributions.

Technological knowing is the shaping of deliberate understanding of persons guided by the revelations gleaned from the competent use of technologies. In this process, the understanding of the person is magnified through the realities of the data obtained from the technology. The nurse enters the world of the other, knowing them as participants in their care rather than as impersonal objects of care. Although the person's status may change from moment to moment, the person is recognized by the nurse as a dynamic and unpredictable human being. Autonomous robots (ARs) will actively participate in knowing the fullness of the person using its technological capabilities. In time, these capabilities will progress as AGI is expected, with a 90% chance, to exist before the end of this century.

213

Part 3

Mutual Designing is a multidimensional process of knowing persons in which both the nurse and the nursed co-create a mutually fulfilling nursing care process derived from both the nurse's design and that of the person being nursed: taken together and jointly practiced, it becomes nursing. A significant issue with mutual designing is the capability of the machine to participate actively in designing the mutual nursing care process. The legitimacy of this concern is centered on the AI that robots may be endowed with. The probability of the development of ASI as Barrat [5] claims will occur much sooner than expected. Current development of robots with AGI is simply programming into robots the "ability to solve problems, learn, and take effective, human-like action, in a variety of environments".

Autonomous robots with ASI will be "a thousand times more intelligent than the smartest human, and it is solving problems at speeds that are millions, even billions of times faster than a human. The thinking it is doing in one minute is equal to what our all-time champion human thinker could do in many, many lifetimes(p. 9)"[5]. Given this progression of intelligence in autonomous robot machines and assuming that a gradual development of artificial intelligence will be dominant, it is highly likely that mutual designing between human persons and autonomous robots with ASI may be as synchronous as between human persons, since both will equally participate in designing the nursing process of care.

Participative engaging promotes the opportunity for simultaneous practice of shared activities which are crucial to knowing persons. In this engagement, the alternating rhythm of implementation and evaluation occurs when the nurse enters the world of the other, and the shared engagement between the nurse and the one nursed results in continuous knowing. As autonomous robots attain AGI, sophisticated activities become the normative expectation; therefore with ASI, the generative expectation will be much more advanced as compared to when robots only had AGI. The participative engagement between human persons and Autonomous Robots will continuously advance as AI progresses to a level that complements the emergence of superintelligent machines and human persons.

Chapter XIII

5. The future of nursing with persons and intelligent machines

In the not-so-distant future, evolving dimensions of science and technology will force the exponential developments of technologies in human healthcare, and the advent of the Singularity (Kurzweil, 2005) [3], i.e. the merging of robotic technologies and ASI (Barrat, 2013) [5], will feature human-robot interactions which will eventually become a seamless engagement with the nurse and nursed as unrecognizable protagonists – to the point where whoever is the machine or human will be unrecognizable. Perhaps it will be Turing's test (1951) [4] that will eventually vindicate the concerns of human beings about "being with" human nurse robots, and successfully support, affirm, and celebrate the humanness of such remarkably evolved human persons in a highly demanding technological world.

Nursing is a transactional engagement between and among human persons. This engagement can be the nursing activities within a space of togetherness that Holopainen (2014) [17] calls a caring encounter. This encounter is similar to Locsin's (2016) [18] technological encounter. As these futuristic practice engagements occur with highly intelligent machines, nursing will require an adaptive view of its practice. Tanioka's (2017) [16] Transactive Relationship Theory of Nursing (TRETON) is a theoretical perspective designed to meet this requirement. Practicing nursing grounded on this theory addresses nursing as a *technological engagement* and *mutual engagement* between the nurse and the person being nursed. The future definition of persons is expected to evolve from the usually represented human beings towards beings such as cybernetic organisms (cyborgs) capable of surviving, living, and being persons in a technologically demanding future world.

With the acceptance of humanoid nurse robots (Ito, et al., 2015) [6] into the field and the constitution of human persons and intelligent machines, the practice of nursing as knowing persons as caring becomes a critical mandate towards recognizing and appreciating persons as participants in their care rather than objects of care. The theory of *Technological Competency as Caring in Nursing* (Locsin,

215

Part 3

2005) [13] acknowledges the practice process of nursing as knowing persons as caring. In this process, the shared events of *technological knowing, mutual designing,* and *participative engaging* (Locsin, 2015) [18] constitute the practice of nursing. As one of these process events is *mutual designing* between human persons and intelligent machines, the challenge becomes overwhelming and complicated. With ASI, the HNRs and human persons will experience mutual engagement (Tanioka 2017) [16]. The characteristic humanness of persons can be realized with the help of this functionality.

The Challenge of Practice

However, in the future, one challenge in this process of nursing can arise in the shared event of mutual designing. Between human persons, this event can be assumed and realized easily and without uncertainties; but when intelligent machines become the "other" in the shared encounter, how will this "process" unfold, and will the assumed "mutuality" occur? Nursing care between human persons and intelligent machines will be realities, and this encounter in mutual designing will materialize. With ASI, HNRs and human persons will experience *mutual engagement* (Tanioka, 2017) [16], thereby expressing communal appreciation in the designing of nursing care. The human nurse robot and the human person can mutually design their nursing care.

The practice of nursing grounded in the science of caring is expressed in the technological competency of nurses in which the dynamic process events of *technological knowing, mutual designing,* and *participative engaging* allow for knowing of persons. This process of knowing persons in the context of nursing embraces the futuristic visioning of engagements between wholly human persons and those who may be endowed with technological enhancers (Locsin, 2016 – Transformative healthcare presentation) [19]. The advancing technologies affecting human persons and those humans with technological enhancements are affirmations of the coexistence of technology and caring unfolding in the process of knowing persons.

216

Chapter XIII

6. Knowledge development through advancing nursing research

This is the future of nursing research within the *Technological Competency as Caring in Nursing* (Locsin, 2005) [13] theory. It articulates "mutual designing" in knowing persons in terms of caring that will challenge future nurse researchers to understand nursing in the context of knowing persons – in terms of caring – and so help future nurses put it into practice effectively.

· Integration of technological competency in the practice of nursing through the nurses' proficient use of advanced technologies.

In situations such as this the imminent coexistence of technology and caring is premised on the affirmation of an informed practice engagement. Such an engagement is focused on technologies of care, with technological competency being integral to the realization of nursing practice as critical to human care.

· Participation in research and development of technologies that recognize nursing as increasingly vital to human care.

The development of nursing knowledge is predicated on the science of nursing from where the scientific evidence supporting nursing activities and futuristic endeavors influencing human caring is derived.

·Engagement in efficient nursing practices involving predictive interventions in human caring, in which human thinking becomes the dynamic through which human persons and intelligent machine can interface.

7. Summary and conclusion

Nursing transpires as the mindful sharing of the experience of persons living their lives meaningfully – these lives being the lives of the nurse and the person being nursed.

Nursing is a uniquely human service for human beings who are served by – not controlled by – human technological creations. Maintaining the influence of

217

Part 3

technological competency within the complex world of nursing is critical to sustaining a mutually rewarding engagement between the nurse and the one nursed.

The coexistence of technology and caring in nursing is exemplified in the characteristics of ARs and human persons. ARs represent extant and advancing technologies endowed with AI, while human persons are caring persons characterized by humanness. For the continuance of human existence, ensuring a high quality of human healthcare is viewed as dependent upon the fundamental provision of technological competency and caring in nursing. Theory-based nursing practice is essential if nursing care practice is to be distinct and to be acknowledged as the contributing factor to human caring, particularly with advanced technologies assuming the indispensable practice process within the science of caring in nursing.

However, with nurse robots having hearts and minds necessarily endowed with AI, they need the ability to observe patients' emotions such as suffering, joy, anguish, or hope. These intelligent machines must be able to appreciate and communicate accurately and appropriately with patients in verbal ways that both human persons and robots can understand.

Nonetheless, there will exist issues of the functionality and ethical use of robot nurses. Furthermore, these issues and problems of having high-level robot nurses will focus on the question of the people to be held accountable for these highly intelligent machines, including their management. Should low-level robot activities such as task completion be considered nursing? Or are these simply healthcare skills or techniques, thus not really falling under the umbrella of the term "nursing"? But what about mid- or higher-level robots which may be able to perform low-level task-completion activities and are programmed with minimal capabilities for human interaction – should human nurses consider these robots partners, or simply as intelligent machine helpers?

When the capacity of ASI machines surpass or transcend human beings, will Tanioka's (2017) [16] question about the prospect of superintelligent robots becoming the human nurses' supervising robots or individual "bosses" become the ultimate consideration for continuing to employ human nurses in the future?

218

Chapter XIII

8. Acknowledgment

I would like to acknowledge Prof. Tetsuya Tanioka's contribution to the development of the manuscript, particularly on the futuristic arguments regarding robot nurses and their role in a practice of nursing that are guided by his theory, TRETON [16].

Acknowledgment is also due to the use of content from the recent publications of Rozzano C. Locsin in both the *Shikoku Acta Medica* and the *Journal of Medical Investigation* where the topics of human caring and the practice of nursing with intelligent machines are articulated and described. The citations follow:

Locsin RC. The Theory of Technological Competency as Caring in Nursing: Guiding Nursing and Health Care. *Shikoku Acta Medica*, Vol. 72, No. 5-6, pp. 163-170, 2016.

Locsin RC. The Co-Existence of Technology and Caring in the Theory of Technological Competency as Caring in Nursing. *Journal of Medical Investigation*, Vol. 64, No. 1-2, pp. 160-164, 2017.

References

[1] Asimov I: The Laws of Robotics, [1970/2012] Reprinted in Asimov, I. Robot. Visions. New York, 1991.

[2] Mori M (K. F. MacDorman & Norri Kageki, Trans.): The Uncanny Valley. IEEE Robotics and Automation, Vol. 19, No. 2, pp. 98-100, 2012.
DOI: 10.1109/MRA.2012.2192811

[3] Kurzweil R: The Singularity is Near: When Humans Transcend Biology. The Penguin Book, New York, NY, 2005.

[4] Turing A: Computing machinery and intelligence. Mind, Vol. 59, pp. 433-460, 1950. http://www.loebner.net/Prizef/TuringArticle.html

[5] Barrat J: Our Final Invention. Thomas Dunne Books, St. Martin's Griffin Press, New York, pp. 9-31, 2013.

219

Part 3

[6] Ito H, Miyagawa M, Kuwamura Y, Yasuhara Y, Tanioka T, Locsin RC: Professional Nurses' Attitudes towards the introduction of Humanoid Nursing Robots (HNRs) in Health Care Settings. Journal of Nursing and Health Sciences, pp. 73-81. 2015.

[7] Watson J: Human Caring Science. Theory of Nursing, p. 22, 2012.

[8] Mayeroff M: On Caring. Harper, Co., New York, 1977.

[9] Roach S: Caring: The Human Mode of Being. Canadian Hospital Association, Toronto, Canada.1987.

[10] Boykin A, Schoenhofer S: Nursing as caring: A model for transforming practice. Sudbury, MA: Jones & Bartlett, 2001.

[11] Locsin RC: The Theory of Technological Competency as Caring in Nursing: Guiding Nursing and Health Care. Shikoku Acta Medica, Vol. 72, No. 5-6, pp. 163-170, 2016.

[12] Bishop AH, Scudder JR: Nursing as a practice rather than an art and a science. Nursing Outlook, Vol. 45, No. 2, pp. 82-85, 1997.

[13] Locsin RC: Technological Competency as Caring in Nursing: A Model for Practice. Sigma Theta Tau International Honor Society of Nursing Press, Indianapolis, IN, 2005.

[14] Locsin RC: The Co-Existence of Technology and Caring in the Theory of Technological Competency as Caring in Nursing. Journal of Medical Investigation. anticipated publication on February, 2017.

[15] Locsin RC: 'Painting a Clear Picture': Technological knowing as contemporary process of nursing. In Locsin, R & Purnell. A Contemporary Process of Nursing: The (Un) Bearable Weight of Knowing Persons in Nursing. Springer Publishing, New York, 2009.

[16] Tanioka T: The Development of the Transactive Relationship Theory of Nursing (TRETON): A Nursing Engagement Model for persons and Robots and Humanoid Nursing Robots. Int J Nurs Clin Pract, Vol. 4, IJNCP-223, 2017. DOI: 10.15344/2394-4978/2017/223

[17] Holopainen G, Kasen A, Nystrom L: The space of togetherness – a caring encounter. Scandinavian Journal of Caring Sciences, Vol. 28, pp. 186-192, 2014.

Chapter XIII

[18] Locsin RC: Technological Competency as Caring in Nursing: Co-creating Moments in Nursing Occurring Within the Universal Technological Domain. The Journal of Theory Construction and Testing, Vol. 20, No. 1, pp. 5-11, 2016.

[19] Locsin RC: Transformative Healthcare Practice Grounded in the Theory of Technological Competency as Caring in Nursing. Keynote Presentation. Third International Health Congress, St. Paul University Philippines, Tuguegarao, Cagayan Valley, Philippines, December 6-7, 2016.

Abstract

This chapter describes the potential developmental issues in the configuration of humanoid healthcare robots for future nursing practice. What distinctive characteristics should humanoid healthcare robots possess, considering nursing care practice? What characteristics are useful for developers of humanoid healthcare robots?

Key Words: Humanoid healthcare robots, Potential developmental issues, Nursing care, Artificial intelligence, Humanoid healthcare robots and human relationships

Chapter XIV

Potential Developmental Issues in the Configuration of

"Nursing" in Humanoid Healthcare Robots

By Tetsuya Tanioka, Rozzano C. Locsin

Chapter XIV

1. Introduction

In order for healthcare robots to understand and communicate with human persons, robots have to be introduced to the world of human healthcare [1]. In this environment of patients in healthcare institutions, valuing proficiency as a characteristic function of healthcare robots demands the realization of healthcare efficiency [2]. Yet, human persons (patients) maintain that it is their right to decide about efficient treatments and healthcare [3]. While this may be so today, in the future patients would have to make a more critical decision, which is whether or not nurses should be allowed to collect and store personal information to know who they are as persons. Further to this is the more unsettling demand that in the future, healthcare robots – in addition to nurses – may be collecting other personal information as well. In order for healthcare robots to be in the world of those they are demanded to care for, robots may need to obtain consent from patients and other medical team members to collect and store life-related information which may be critical to human caring. However, forms of consent can be implied or obtained through hardcopies by robots through their integrated language which may include affirming protocols.

The reason it is necessary to obtain consent from the patient is to establish the capability of human nurses – whether they are proficient "enough" – to care for them even before they build a confidential relationship with them [4]. This relationship refers to that between human nurses and patients. Therefore, that human persons and nurses view healthcare robots as trustworthy requires a response to the question, "What is required of humanoid robots in order to establish a trusting relationship between them and human persons?"

First, if a nurse does not have logical thinking abilities, it is inarguable that engineers or business giants would take the initiative to produce healthcare robots, with capabilities following only their perceived attention to healthcare as generally that of task completion. If this is prevented, then humanoid robots may be designed and developed following a nursing perspective in which the expected outcome is not

223

Part 3

limited only to task completion. Moreover, with the possibility of the government granting licenses to healthcare robots, these robots may or will be attributed some collegial "respect" by nurses and co-health care professionals who work at hospitals.

Second, introducing healthcare robots can have ethical problems. For example, in the case of human nurses, there is a standard of safe patient care concerning their technical abilities and critical attention to privacy that is set up through licensing. However, for the moment, there is nothing similar to that standard for healthcare robots.

Nurses must think about how the tasks should be dealt with if and when the healthcare robots start performing the same tasks. The consequence of programmed or automatic task programming increases precision and risk of unsatisfactory performance of care.

Since healthcare robots are none other than personalized artificial intelligence (AI) machines, their capabilities might be expected to fall below the level of human persons. As such, it is natural that human persons should consider them as assistants to nurses. However, in the future some robots with enhanced AI may have the ability to improve themselves through experiences just as human beings do. Owing to this, it is possible that robots with AI will exceed human capabilities when advancements in science will bring about AI with high functioning learning capabilities [5]. In that case, the problem of healthcare robots taking nursing initiatives over human nurses might possibly occur sometime in the future.

Additionally, other uses of robots with AI can be for purposes other than healthcare. It is important to realize and recognize that without nurses' influence on the development of Robots with AI, this development toward purposes beyond healthcare cannot be stopped, and that these types of robots may in the future be utilized as "completer of healthcare tasks" or a type of rescue robots instead.

224

Chapter XIV

2. Ethics and healthcare robots

These days, ethical thinking has been spreading in hospitals. Ethics – as discussed in a lot of research, new treatments, and clinical examinations of new drugs – has become a cornerstone in the development and assurance of scientific research, one that is rigorous and worthy of scientific dissemination [6]. However, presently, the development of humanoid robots with artificial intelligence and the research into their usefulness in healthcare are progressing well only under the initiative of the robot and healthcare development companies or those who can profit from these robots in the market.

It was taken for granted in Japanese society that advertisements presenting the relationships of humanlike robots and human beings are constantly shown on TV or the internet. This makes the idea of using robots in elderly care seem to be commonplace. From an economic perspective, the government and many companies have invested huge amounts of money into robotics research. From an everyday perspective, families are looking for ways to facilitate the care of their aging relatives [7]. On the other hand, in nursing care facilities (especially for the elderly), healthcare robots help the elderly simply by transferring or moving them around. These have already been developed by engineers and are currently being advertised for sale [8].

Assuming that these robots can be introduced into ordinary homes as AI-equipped humanoid robots for household use, it would still be difficult to investigate their use and value in ordinary homes given that ethics committees in hospitals respond to the prospect with a narrow sense of ethical values [9, 10]. Moreover, hospitals might encounter a situation where a number of healthcare robots are introduced without the Hospital Administrators knowing about it at all. When Robots with AI are introduced for nursing, the nurse may consider if these robots must come as naturally humanlike or not. Unless nurses know what the Robot with AI is and its capabilities, future nurses cannot assume the kinds of problems which may occur when using robots for nursing. Modern healthcare is strongly connected

225

Part 3

with technology and auxiliary medical services are put in place via technology. Technology is indispensable for healthcare; therefore, in order to provide the best quality of nursing care, it is necessary to consider the relationship between medicine, nursing, and technology.

2.1. Abilities required of healthcare robots to engage in nursing care

Anthropomorphic machines are embodied mechanical entities interacting with humans [11]. For one such machine, the proper sharing in and of patient experiences is contingent upon the following abilities: most critical of them being the ability to remember; the ability to process language and maintain a conversation; and the ability to read and illustrate emotions from facial expressions. All of these will become necessary functions for healthcare robots. Furthermore, in healthcare settings, it is necessary to facilitate and encourage conversations centering on the relationship between "human" and "human" as well as conversations between "human" and "robot" and eventually among "human" to "human" and to "robot".

Nurses are required to have the ability to understand patients; therefore, if robots are to practice nursing, they may be required to have high-level thinking properties/processes such as those of sympathy, confidence, and conscience necessary to engage in a nursing situation [12]. In essence, the seeming sentience that robots with AI can express and appreciate are critical to the achievement of humanlike features including the demonstration of the five senses and humanlike memory abilities [13, 14]. Importantly, Robots with AI ought to exhibit the abilities of expressing emotions – with all the requisite characteristics – for them to be considered as practicing nursing. What is applicable from the human mind is the ability to express emotions and "mind" [15]. In order for Robots with AI to function as humanlike as possible, at the level of nursing professionals, the robots need to understand patients, demonstrate expertise in human caring, and express sympathy and kindness in their daily practice. Moreover, in care-giving relationships with patients, not only the patients but also the nurses need to grow.

226

What does the human nurse's ability to grow as caregivers mean for Robots with AI?

Human nurses learn from their patients through shared experiences [16]. For this reason, before robots can practice nursing, it is necessary to develop their AI – assuming that healthcare robots can record and store empirical knowledge into their databases – and be able to share perceived difficulties with patients. While robots with AI are equipped with learning functions, it is necessary to define what, how far, and how AI should learn. Furthermore, the effectiveness of the AI's learning becomes the most important issue, because an AI's learning ability is considered to be basically different from that of humans who can learn anything through experience or study (although sometimes inefficiently). Therefore, based on modern AI's learning abilities, it is important to define what, how far, and how healthcare robots can study in advance and simulate learning systems for their future development.

2.2. Nursing care, Robots with AI, and human relationships

It is necessary to provide nursing care "when necessary and successfully" in interactive relationships with patients. Nursing care is a responsibility for the person and for others. In order to convey this sense of responsibility to others, it should be a real responsibility [17, 18]. In other words, healthcare robots should have the ability of becoming wholeheartedly involved with others.

Conventional nursing has been focused on human relationships. According to Travelbee's model [19], nursing is accomplished through relationships between humans beginning with an original encounter and then progressing through stages of emerging identities, developing feelings of empathy and sympathy. The nurse and patient establish a rapport in the final stage. Meeting the nursing goals requires the creation of a genuine human-to-human relationship, which can only be established by an interaction process.

In the practice of nursing, knowing is the essential process that initiates the relationship between the nurse and nursed. Carper [20] has described four

Part 3

fundamental patterns of ways of knowing in nursing. Knowing the other person continually and intentionally leads to understanding the person more fully as a person. All persons have many aspects which change from moment to moment. Therefore, healthcare robots have to use the process of "knowing" to understand the person in the moment.

Nurses need to reflect on the nurse-caring process and consider how to provide even better care so they can realize the care receivers' hopes, dreams, and aspirations; or help them grow while they are under treatments [21]. For this purpose, elderly patients are asked what they most currently desire. Robots with AI are expected to compile the rich descriptions of the nurses' experiences in a database. Moreover, other personal information – including photographs related to their past experiences from their families, for example – are then inserted as information into the robots' database. Through this process, the conversations between elderly patients and healthcare robots – in which individual characters are more emphasized – can be deepened; healthcare robots and the patients they care for share their lives fully through talking about the experiences of their illnesses so the patients could feel good. In this sense, it is important to program Robots with AI from the perspective of fostering an interactive relationship between machine and human. The following features assume explanatory and structural roles and actions towards understanding and appreciating Robots with AI and the endeavor towards maintaining humanness.

Humans grow by giving or receiving care. The robots should have the function of memorizing what care receivers talk about so the healthcare robots would be able to enhance their conversation ability as a function of nursing care.

The robots should have the function of conveying empathic understanding, or the capability of expressing emotion, so they could sympathize with care receivers.

The robots should not have intimidating appearances so that the care receivers would feel able to trust them.

228

Chapter XIV

The robots should be programmed for conversation and other nonverbal behavior so they could accurately deliver their intentions and then their compassionate care.

Nevertheless, the development of computer-human interfacing, with practitioner programming, is required before the healthcare robots could function within the transactive relationship model [22]. In combination, a Robot with AI needs sensory mechanisms that share the four aforementioned features with caregivers and other members of the healthcare teams. Healthcare robot utilization, particularly in elderly care settings, is therefore projected in the near future. With enhancements in AI, basic questions will change, particularly the issue of whether or not healthcare robots and human care will ultimately be undifferentiated.

2.2.1. What is a healthcare robot?

Humanoid robots programmed as healthcare robots are projected to be loaded with artificial brains possessing super AI by 2050. With these capabilities, humanoid robots can now know human persons, cooperate with nurses and healthcare professionals, and may be able to share experiences.

2.2.2. When will healthcare robots be introduced to elderly institutions or hospitals?

The use of robotic technology is strongly desired to relieve the burden of nursing-care workers. However, because of market, safety, and practical issues, nursing equipment that uses advanced technologies is going through a slow development [23]. Initially used in research with the purpose of understanding the human body in detail and eventually sourcing motion and control solutions already engineered by nature, humanoid robots are becoming increasingly present in our lives [23]. For such robots, clinical trials have measured their effects on the elderly, and perhaps by 2020 some of these robots will be introduced to hospitals and facilities. For example, "Pepper©", from Softbank Corporation, was leased to

229

Part 3

individuals in Japan in 2015, and in 2016 "Pepper©" was made available for commercial use in facilities, e.g. hospitals.

2.2.3. Who will work with healthcare robots and where?

Healthcare robots will function "in cooperation" with nurses and healthcare professionals in settings where their functional characteristics will be greatly required or needed, such as in hospitals, elderly care facilities, and outpatient clinics or physicians' offices and clinics. Furthermore, there is a human resource problem stemming from Japan having the highest life expectancy in the world today – more than any other country. The idea is to build healthcare robots that will promote the quality of nursing care and support people in hospitals, care facilities, and homes.

2.3. Nurses' role and interdisciplinary teamwork

It is necessary to re-envision the description of aspects of the nursing metaparadigm of person, nursing, health, and environment [24-26]. Persons can be understood as healthcare providers, or nurses; or in the future, healthcare robots, or humanoid robots. The end focus includes nursing expressions of caring in which the nurse and the nursed enhance the living of the latter. While early healthcare robots may do the job of nursing assistants well, their advancing performance is going to improve by the evolution of computers and AI, thereby enhancing their performance and mechanical functional levels. There will be a marked difference between healthcare robots and Humanoid Nurse Robots (HNRs) [27].

Therefore, knowing patient and family situations through healthcare robot assessment, and sharing patient information with an interdisciplinary team will become essential health and nursing care demands. In addition, healthcare robots can help patients physically move around or they can perform simple healthcare tasks like taking vital signs or delivering medicines and recording of medical/nursing records; they can also provide information to the nurses and other healthcare professionals. These simple tasks will be expected, but in addition, healthcare robots will also be expected to engage in knowing activities, much like in

230

Chapter XIV

current physical assessments, using more technologically advanced instruments. The healthcare robot will be evolving and eventually engaging in conversation, and other interactive activities. A transactive relation will ensue, guided by Tanioka's (2017) Transactive Relationship Theory of Nursing (TRETON) [22]; the evolution of nursing engagement via technological encounter will come into reality.

By 2020, the facilities for elderly care and hospital settings will have healthcare robots. The development of databases on interactions between healthcare robots and elderly patients for use in elderly facilities will proceed through the combination of database content and recreation services for the elderly, more than in the realm of human services. In 2025, the role of healthcare robots will advance into capabilities of discourse, such abilities corresponding to the license of a human nurse, in consideration of ethical issues. Researchers and humanoid robot engineers will develop the Nurse Robot Caring Database (NRDB). The performance of robot development based on the NRDB will be considered by nurse researchers and other medical staff as critical information. By 2030, a better process of healthcare robots knowing patients will have been developed which will advance the practical application of interactive features of healthcare robots on understanding patient conditions. Sentience becomes possible and a more transactive healthcare robot will be put into "practice". In 2050, the Singularity will have been realized and healthcare robots may be able to transcend their artificial intelligence. Standards of ethics and performance of healthcare robots will be instituted and their practice will need certification from the national government; and possibly, licensure will be mandatory to ensure both human and robot safety. Problems with robot technicalities will be at the minimum, thereby assuring a safer robot care performance.

There will be no limitation to the scope of activities in the performance of the robot, since the fuel cells that power robots will be greatly enhanced. As healthcare robots become essential to the interdisciplinary team care, and they start to perform activities involving knowing patients, healthcare robots might be able to play a significant and valuable role to medical and welfare teams. The increasing quality of nursing care, knowing patient experiences, quality of caring in nursing, satisfaction

231

Part 3

of nurse and nursed, and the patient's quality of health and wellbeing are all pertinent expectations and functions that healthcare robots can fundamentally perform as a legitimate member of the healthcare team.

3. Conclusion

The main question still remains: Do nursing activities and their completion make nursing care nursing? Will the design and development of a healthcare robot aided by contemporary and future advancements exponentially improve, thereby providing opportunities for human care that may likely rival that of human nurses? When these functions are achieved, healthcare robots will outgrow their expected task-oriented care practices and engage in more nursing care activities much like a human nurse can – they will engage in transactive relationships, thus enabling a care receiver to live his life meaningfully.

Can a robot be a "nurse" or is it merely a healthcare robot? If nursing care activities will be expected of these "nurse robots", will a registered nurse's license be required for robots to engage in "nursing practice?" Ray Kurzweil [5] has predicted that the technological singularity will occur in 2045, when artificial intelligences surpass human beings as the smartest and most capable life forms on the Earth. While it may be assumed that nursing is an engagement that involves higher cognitive functions, healthcare robots will eventually become technologically advanced enough that they effectively become nurse robots that meet the essential elements of nursing practice.

A critical ethical issue remains. While there is a Code of Ethics in the United States of America that guides healthcare and nursing practice, the ultimate question is, "Who will supervise the performance of tasks of healthcare robots?"

Robot development for medical, nursing, and welfare care is progressing well, but one thing is certain: The legal development supporting its practice needs to advance in congruence with *advancements* in robot, AI technologies, and *human beings*.

Chapter XIV

References

[1] Huston C: The Impact of Emerging Technology on Nursing Care: Warp Speed Ahead. The Online Journal of Issues in Nursing, Vol. 18, No. 2, Manuscript 1, 2013. DOI: 10.3912/OJIN.Vol18No02Man01

[2] Robotic Online, Tanya MA: Robots and Healthcare Saving Lives Together. Robotic Industries Association.
http://www.robotics.org/content-detail.cfm/Industrial-Robotics-Industry-Insights/R obots-and-Healthcare-Saving-Lives-Together/content_id/5819
(Accessed 27 November 2016)

[3] Goold SD, Lipkin M: The Doctor–Patient Relationship: Challenges, Opportunities, and Strategies. Journal of General Internal Medicine, Vol. 14, Supplement 1, pp. S26-S33, 1999. DOI: 10.1046/j.1525-1497.1999.00267.x

[4] McParland J, Scott PA, Arndt M, Dassen T, Gasull M, Lemonidou C, Valimaki M, Leino-Kilpi H: Autonomy and clinical practice. 2: Patient privacy and nursing practice. Br J Nurs, Vol. 9, No. 9, pp. 566-569, 2000.
DOI: 10.12968/bjon.2000.9.9.6293

[5] Kurzweil R: The Singularity Is Near: When Humans Transcend Biology. Viking Books, New York, 2005.

[6] Novossiolova T, Sture J: Towards the responsible conduct of scientific research: is ethics education enough? Medicine Conflict and Survival, Vol. 28, No. 1, pp. 73-84, 2012.

[7] Rathmann M, Care Robots for an Over-Aging Society: A Technical Solution for Japan's Demographic Problem?
http://www.kuasu.cpier.kyoto-u.ac.jp/wp-content/uploads/2015/10/Care-Robot s-for-an-Over-Aging-Society.pdf (Acsseced 27 November 2016)

[8] Smashing Robotics, Thirteen Advanced Humanoid Robots for Sale Today.
https://www.smashingrobotics.com/thirteen-advanced-humanoid-robots-for-sal e-today/

[9] Ito H, Yasuhara Y, Tanioka, Locsin RC: Adoption of medical/welfare robots in medical environments and its ethical issues. Proceedings of 8th International

233

Conference on Natural Language Processing and Knowledge Engineering (NLP-KE'12), pp. 560-562, China, Sep. 2012.

[10] Fuji S, Ito H, Yasuhara Y, Shihong H, Tanioka T, Locsin RC: Discussion of Nursing Robot's Capability and Ethical Issues. Information : an International Interdisciplinary Journal, Vol. 17, No. 1, pp. 349-354, 2014.

[11] Locsin RC, Tanioka T, Kawanishi C: Anthropomorphic Machines and the Practice of Nursing: Knowing Persons as Whole in the Moment. Proceedings of 2005 IEEE International Conference on Natural Language Processing and Knowledge Engineering, pp. 825-829, 2005. DOI: 10.1109/NLPKE.2005.1598850

[12] Boykin A, Schoenhofer S: Nursing as caring: A model for transforming practice. Sudbury, MA: Jones & Bartlett, 2001.

[13] Bar-Cohen Y: The progress in human-like robots towards having them in every home and business. Int J Adv Robot Syst, Vol. 12, Supplement 1, pp. 55-67, 2015.

[14] Pino M, Boulay M, Jouen F, Rigaud AS: Are we ready for robots that care for us? Attitudes and opinions of older adults toward socially assistive robots. Frontiers in Aging Neuroscience, Vol. 7, 141, 2015. DOI: 10.3389/fnagi.2015.00141

[15] Yasuhara Y, Tamayama C, Kikukawa K, Osaka K, Tanioka T, Watanabe N, Chiba S, Miyoshi M, Locsin RC, Ren F, Fuji S, Ogasawara H, Mifune K: Required Function of the Caring Robot with Dialogue Ability for Patients with Dementia. AIA International Advanced Information Institute, Vol. 4, No. 1, pp. 31-42, 2012.

[16] Rørtveit K, Sætre HB, Leiknes I, Joa I, Testad I, Severinsson E: Patients' Experiences of Trust in the Patient-Nurse Relationship – A Systematic Review of Qualitative Studies. Open Journal of Nursing, Vol. 5, pp. 195-209, 2015. DOI: 10.4236/ojn.2015.53024.

[17] Mitchell PH: Defining Patient Safety and Quality Care. In: Hughes RG, editor. Patient Safety and Quality: An Evidence-Based Handbook for Nurses. Rockville (MD): Agency for Healthcare Research and Quality (US), Chapter 1, 2008. Available from: https://www.ncbi.nlm.nih.gov/books/NBK2681/

[18] Izumi S: Quality improvement in nursing: Administrative mandate or professional responsibility? Nursing Forum, Vol. 47, No. 4, pp. 260-267, 2012.
DOI: http://doi.org/10.1111/j.1744-6198.2012.00283.x

[19] Travelbee J: Interpersonal aspects of nursing. Philadelphia: F.A. Davis, 1966.

[20] Carper BA: Fundamental Patterns of Knowing in Nursing. Advances in Nursing Science, Vol. 1, No. 1, pp. 13-24, 1978.

[21] Smith S, James A, Brogan A, Adamson E, Gentleman M: Reflections about experiences of compassionate care from award winning undergraduate nurses – What, so what … now what?. Journal of Compassionate Health Care, Vol. 3, No. 1, pp. 1-11, 2016.

[22] Tanioka T: The Development of the Transactive Relationship Theory of Nursing (TRETON): A Nursing Engagement Model for persons and Robots and Humanoid Nursing Robots. Int J Nurs Clin Pract, Vol. 4, IJNCP-223, 2017.
DOI: 10.15344/2394-4978/2017/223

[23] Robotic Devices for Nursing Care Project, Robotic Care Devices Portal. http://robotcare.jp/?lang=en

[24] Fawcett J: Theory: basis for the study and practice of nursing education. Journal of Nursing Education, Vol. 24, No. 6, pp. 226-229, 1985.
http://www.slackjournals.com/jne

[25] Fawcett J: On the requirements for a metaparadigm: an invitation to dialogue. Nursing Science Quarterly, vol. 9, No. 3, pp. 94-97, 1996.
DOI:10.1177/089431849600900305

[26] Fawcett J: The Metaparadigm of Nursing: Present Status and Future Refinements. The Journal of Nursing Scholarship, Vol. 16, No. 3, pp. 84-87, 1984.
DOI: 10.1111/j.1547-5069.1984.tb01393.x

[27] Ito H, Miyagawa M, Kuwamura Y, Yasuhara Y, Tanioka T, Locsin RC: Professional Nurses' Attitudes towards the Introduction of Humanoid Nurse Robots (HNRs) in Health Care Settings. Journal of Nursing and Health Sciences, Vol. 9 (spl Issue), pp. 73-81, 2015.

Epilogue

Tetsuya Tanioka, Rozzano C. Locsin

What is the future of nursing robots in healthcare settings?

It may be that the future of nursing robots depends upon the definition of what comprises nursing and its practice, in which the types of robots and the consequent outcomes of care may be referred. Furthermore, the types of nursing robots deliberated in this book are focused on those of much importance to elderly care. Other than the desire of the authors and editors to illuminate these types of nurse robots, there is also the debate on the ethics and morality of nursing robots in healthcare.

The future of nursing robots can be described as imminent. As technology that makes things efficient, nursing robots for elderly care – in this case referring to the system in a developed country like Japan – are a desired addition to human healthcare. The thematic organization of the book was designed to address current influences on robot technologies in healthcare. Nevertheless, it seems that the envisioned solution may just be the design, development, and utilization of nursing robots. However, how do we use such robots for nursing care and healthcare? Most importantly, the authors and editors are continuing to ask the ultimate question, "Does the contemporary and the future human world with its attendant advanced technologies need humanoid nurse robots (HNRs) for clinical human care situations?"

Technology must always be convenient for humans. If so, the humanoid robot must be useful for human beings. In recent years, humanoid robots have gone on sale in Japan. Whether humans consider robots as useful for human existence depends largely on whether or not these robots can communicate with human users. It is a reality that even if a box-shaped, self-propelled robot is moving in a hospital, it is simply recognized to be "just a robot".

Epilogue

However, these humanoid nurse robots need to have highly "evolved" communication skills in order for patients and nurses to recognize them, if not as "like persons", then at least as personified and anthropomorphic machines.

Healthcare robots (HRs) that can perform simple tasks like taking vital signs or performing precise delivery [1], for example, of medications are critically needed. Reducing these types of human-dependent activities will provide human nurses space to focus on more important tasks – for example, on direct human caring relationships and nursing care for these patients. Furthermore, healthcare robot research [2] urgently needs to focus on developing new computational algorithms for determining accurate patient emotional state classification in interactions between human and intelligent machine during healthcare services.

Any HNR designed to "replace" or enhance the work of the human nurse and to increase patient satisfaction must be cognizant of this relationality [3]. In this way, it behooves researchers of Computer Science, Robotics, and Engineering to obtain an increased appreciation for the value of nursing care practices in healthcare, to realize hints from the information and recommendations provided, and to gain the ability to design and create a new robot technology to support nursing practice. Therefore, in order to make the humanoid robot perform nursing, it requires advanced performance of real-time nursing. Self-aware robots may be construed as the ideal HNRs.

We define the Humanoid Nursing Robots as:

(1) Autonomous robots [4], or intelligent machines capable of performing tasks in the world by themselves, without explicit human control. Examples range from autonomous helicopters to Roomba, the robot vacuum cleaner;

(2) HRs [5], or robots used in the healthcare setting. HRs can be used in healthcare settings, but it does not retain the competency of "caring in nursing" of the human nurse. Low-level humanoid robot nurses are categorized as HRs;

Epilogue

(3) Humanoid nurse robot (HNR), or fully functional robotic nurses who can do the same job as human nurses, including true and genuine nursing care for human beings.

Following the evolution process from HRs to HNRs shows a real possibility of perfecting "real" HRs and HNRs in the future [6], those that can assist with the demands of human caring in nursing, especially among older adults with dementia.

Level 1: HRs in 2020. These robots are projected to be low level "robots" that work much like an HNR does. This intelligent machine will do vital sign measurements: blood pressure, pulse measurement, SPO_2 measurement, clerking, and so on. It is this public image of the nurse particularly in hospital settings that provides a semblance of its ontological and epistemological work. Activities such as these can include bathing, feeding, taking vital signs, making beds, assisting physicians, etc.

Level 2: HRs in 2030. This type of robot can manage and perform moderate-level work. The HNR is a robot capable of interpersonal communication, and – in addition to the expected work of low level nurses – can understand, empathize, and sympathize with patients and families. Robot nurses at this level can also interact with other professionals. It may seem inconceivable that this so called "excellent nursing" practice should be the outcome of competency of practice in human engagement involving physico-physiological and interactive relations with and among other persons as patients. If we are to make the nurse robot's heart/mind compatible with artificial intelligence (AI) – assisted nursing, we need to build into the robot the ability to first observe the patient's suffering, correctly evaluate it, and then communicate its findings to the patient in appropriate words. Also, nurse robots communicate their empathetic connections with technological competence. For example, actions that integrate not only words but also "knowledge, judgment, technical skills, and care" are expected of these nursing robots.

Level 3: HNRs in 2040. These robots will be expected to perform high-level work as the HNR assumes the role of a fully functional robotic nurse who can do the

Epilogue

same job as a human nurse. It is important to be reminded that all levels of robot nurses are equipped with terminals of electronic medical charts for easy access.

Level 4: Humanoid nurse robot in 2050. By this time, transcendence will have become the main feature of robot functionality. It refers to the moment when AI finally exceeds human intelligence and physical functioning. Should we aim to develop the HNR towards transcendence?

This transcendence is a result of the Singularity [7], a hypothetical event in the far future when AI and other technologies have become so advanced that humanity undergoes a dramatic and irreversible change – this may be a hoped-for occasion in some quarters. Many definitions of Singularity exist, but one that serves AI and humanity well is Kurzweil's description. Singularity [8] refers to a trait marking one as distinct from others – a peculiarity. Often, computers can manage to illustrate a hypothetical point in the far future when AI will surpass human intelligence and gain the ability to self-replicate and improve itself autonomously. The Singularity must lead to an HNR-enriched human society, and we have to share the benefits to the rest of the world for global social growth.

As the demands and needs for quality healthcare rise – particularly in human-resource poor environments and among the older adult population – the utilization of human-machine process requirements are intensified, and the realities and consequences of transactive relationships have become integral to assuring quality human healthcare.

Nursing caring practices involving intelligent machines with highly sophisticated robotic technological functions such as interactive capabilities may be the best option for the care of the increasingly older adult population, particularly those members of the same population afflicted with dementia. In this situation, the HNRs equipped with AI will be programmed to appreciate the meanings of the lived experiences of older adults.

Human caring has always been based on a human-to-human relationship. The realization of human and intelligent machine transactions in healthcare has been the impetus for the development of the Transactive Relationship Theory of Nursing

239

Epilogue

(TRETON) [9]. Especially, in a nonhuman-to-human relationship, as in the case of HNRs, it is essential to consider what is required of them in the aspects of ethical concerns and human safety. Also, if HNRs are to support patients directly, they will be required to have the same level of comprehensive judgment and responsiveness as the human nurses and care staff display in their everyday life. This includes the abilities to deeply observe, judge, quickly respond, and conduct caring with an emphasis on individuality. If HNRs are to support patients independently, abilities close to those of humans will be required of them in addition to the appropriate knowledge and skills to do so.

A low-level robot nurse performs work that should be called non-nursing or as a medical aid assistant no matter who thinks what these technologies can do. However, a higher-level HNR with higher-level artificial intelligence is expected to exceed the capabilities of human beings. Once these higher-level HNRs exceed the capacity of human beings, there will naturally occur the argument of whether or not the robot nurse should now become one's superior or whether or not the robot nurse should remain the subordinate.

References

[1] Huang S, Tanioka T, Locsin RC, Parker M, Masory O: Functions of a caring robot in nursing. Proceedings of 7th International Conference on Natural Language Processing and Knowledge Engineering (NLP-KE '11), pp.425-429, 2011. DOI: 10.1109/NLPKE.2011.6138237

[2] Swangnetr M, David B, Kaber D: Emotional State Classification in Patient – Robot Interaction Using Wavelet Analysis and Statistics-Based Feature Selection. Proceedings of 2013 IEEE Transactions on Human-Machine Systems, Vol. 43, No. 1, pp. 63-75, 2013.

[3] Locsin RC, Tanioka T, Kawanishi C: Anthropomorphic machines and the practice of nursing: knowing persons as whole in the moment. Proceedings of 2005 IEEE International Conference on Natural Language Processing and Knowledge Engineering, IEEE NLP-KE '05, 2005. DOI: 10.1109/NLPKE.2005.1598850

[4]   George BA: Autonomous Robots, From Biological Inspiration to Implementation and Control. MIT press books, 2005.

ISBN-13: 978-0262025782

[5]   Wynsberghe AV: Healthcare Robots: Ethics. Design and Implementation (Emerging Technologies, Ethics and International Affairs), Routledge, 2015.

ISBN-13: 978-1472444332

[6]   Tanioka T, Osaka K, Locsin RC, Yasuhara Y, Ito H: Recommended design and direction of development for Humanoid nurse robots perspective from nursing re-searchers. Intelligent Control and Automation, Vol. 8, No. 2, pp. 96-110, May 26, 2017. DOI: 10.4236/ica.2017.82008

[7]   English Oxford Living Dictionaries: Singularity.

https://en.oxforddictionaries.com/definition/singularity

[8]   The American Heritage® Dictionary of the English Language: 5th edition Copyright 2013 by Houghton Mifflin Harcourt Publishing Company, Published by Houghton Mifflin Harcourt Publishing Company.

[9]   Tanioka T: The Development of the Transactive Relationship Theory of Nursing (TRETON): A Nursing Engagement Model for persons and Robots and Humanoid Nursing Robots. Int J Nurs Clin Pract, Vol. 4, IJNCP-223, 2017.

DOI: 10.15344/2394-4978/2017/223

INDEX

[A, a]

Act on Public Health Nurses, Midwives
 and Nurses 192
Actigraph 53
activities of daily living (ADL) 149
activity assist robot 36
Actroid 119
actuator 72
Aesthetic knowing 183
aging 36
AI (artificial intelligence)
 .... 208, 214, 218, 224, 229
 — -equipped humanoid robots ... 225
 — machines 224
 — /Robot Care System 125
anthropomorphic machines ... 180, 226
artificial general intelligence (AGI) ·210
artificial superintelligence (ASI)
 .... 208, 214
ASIMO 88
autonomous
 — decisions 152
 — robots 214

[B, b]

Bag of Concepts 111

basic components of robots 69
bathing aids 26
BEAR 36, 39
behavioral and psychological symptoms
 of dementia (BPSD) 52
big data 108
Bodyweight Support System 40
BSS 40, 43

[C, c]

CAR 45
care 36
 — assist robot (s) 36, 44, 45
Care Robot Trio 124
caregivers of elderly persons 9
caring 87, 94, 175
 — persons 209
 — , compassion 101
CHI 131
code of ethics for nurses 200
communication 87, 93
 — functions 88
 — robots 116
 — skills 93, 96
communicative robots 88
community-based integrated care

243

Index

systems (CBICS) ·················· 11

comparative cultural knowledge ····· 97

compassion ················· 87, 92, 94

complex multi-dimensional concept　92

computers ····························· 152

connection between technology and
　caring in nursing ·················· 176

conversational robots ··············· 96

conversations ······················· 180

critical ethical issue ················ 232

[D, d]

databases ···························· 227

deep learning ······················· 108

dementia ···························· 96

Dorothy Orem's self-care deficit theory
　································· 149

dynamic nursing process ··········· 212

[E, e]

elderly ······························· 36

— with dementia, the ··············· 8

emotion ······························· 89

— corpus ···························· 111

emotional

— cues ····························· 100

— response ························· 154

empathetic ···················· 88, 89

— expressions ······················· 93

empathic ························· 88, 89

— competence ······················· 99

— relationships ····················· 93

— robots ···························· 100

— understanding ········· 87, 89, 100

empathy ··················· 87, 89, 92, 94

— cycle ····························· 94

Empirical knowing ················· 183

empirical knowledge ··············· 227

Enriching Mental Engineering ····· 118

Economic Partnership Agreement (EPA)
　································· 13

ethical

— challenges ······················· 100

— thinking ························· 225

Ethical knowing ··················· 183

ethics ····························· 225

exercise assist robot (s) ············· 36

expression recognition ·············· 88

[F, f]

Fully-automated general purpose IoT
　type AI/Robot ···················· 133

fundamental patterns of knowing in
　nursing ························· 181

244

Index

[G, g]

GEAR 36, 38

genuine human-to-human relationship

.... 227

GI 126

GPGPU 109

[H, h]

Hasegawa's Dementia Scale-Revised

(HDS-R) 55

healthcare 149, 150

— (nurse) robot (s) 166, 167-170,

172-175, 178-181, 184, 224, 225, 227-

229, 231

— characteristics 179

Heart Rate Variability (HRV) 54

history and definition of robots 69

HSR 45, 46

human

— emotion 116

— persons ... 168, 170-172, 174, 176

— -centered care 158

— -friendly robots 69

— support robot 45

— -robot

— caring practice 97

— relationships 101

— -to-intelligent machine 141

— relationships 173

humanoid

— nurse robots (HNRs) ... 87, 208,

230

— nursing robots 192

— robot program 94

— robots 208, 225, 229

[I, i]

independence assist robot (s) 36, 40

individual dignity 140

indoor mobility aids 25

intelligent machines 172, 208

interaction 100

interdisciplinary collaborative research

.... 101

International Council of Nurses, the

(ICN) 200

International Organization for

Standardization (ISO) 29, 192

internet of things 126

inverted pendulum 39

IoT 126

ISO 29

— 13482 151

— standard 151

245

Index

[J, j]

JIN 131

[K, k]

k-nearest neighbor 111

knowing 228

— person 181

— persons as a practice process of

nursing 212

[L, l]

literature review 88

lived experience of caring 176

Long Short-Term Memory (LSTM) · 109

long-term care insurance system, the

.... 11

low-fidelity robots 88

[M, m]

medical insurance 11

Mental State Transition Network

(MSTN) 117, 119

metaparadigm 230

mirror neuron system 91

mirroring 91

Mobile Servant Robot 29

monitoring systems

— for nursing care homes 27

— for private homes 28

motion recognition 88

Multi-agent small type AI/Robot ··· 131

multidimensional 94

mutual

— designing 212, 214, 216, 217

— engagements 177

— experience 97

[N, n]

neural matching mechanisms 91

New Five Laws for Care Robots user

.... 142

New Robot Strategy, the 60

non-wearable transfer aids 22

NTT Docomo Chat API 109

nurse caring database for the robot, the

(NRDB) 231

nursing 89, 92, 172

— care 149

— encounter (s) ·· 171, 172, 177, 185

— encounters 171, 172

— goals 227

— practice 210

— shortage 158

Nursing as Caring 209

Nursing Robots 69

246

Index

[O, o]

old-fashioned robot ·················· 170

On Caring ························· 175

outdoor mobility aids ················ 23

[P, p]

participative engaging ··· 212, 214, 216

patient's experiences ·················· 180

patient-centered ······················· 93

patients ···························· 168

Pepper ························ 229, 230

personal care

— robotics ························· 150

— robots ·························· 20

Personal Carrier Robot ·············· 29

Personal knowing ·················· 182

person-centered approaches ·········· 96

Physical Assistant Robot ············ 29

programs ························· 100

[Q, q]

quality ··························· 150

— nursing care ···················· 158

[R, r]

receptionists ······················ 88

reciprocal relationship ················ 87

rehabilitation ······················· 36

Ren-CECps ························· 111

Rinna ····························· 109

robot ························· 69, 89

— communication research ········ 87

— engagements in Japan ········· 192

robotic care equipment ··············· 6

robotics ··············· 149, 150, 158, 159

— and nursing ···················· 152

— research ························ 87

Robots with AI ···················· 228

Robovie R-2 ······················· 119

rodeo ····························· 40

Rogers ···························· 87

role of the robot, the ················ 14

[S, s]

sacred

— in nursing ······················ 153

— to nursing ····················· 149

safety

— features ························ 29

— measures ······················ 69

— of robots ······················ 69

— requirements ··················· 29

self-

— awareness ·················· 124, 125

— determination ··················· 152

— understanding ··················· 125

247

Index

sensor ⋯⋯⋯⋯⋯⋯⋯⋯⋯⋯⋯⋯ 71

Seq2Seq ⋯⋯⋯⋯⋯⋯⋯⋯⋯⋯ 109

shared experiences ⋯⋯⋯⋯⋯ 227

SHIN ⋯⋯⋯⋯⋯⋯⋯⋯⋯⋯⋯⋯ 126

simple manual ⋯⋯⋯⋯⋯⋯⋯ 170

singularity ⋯⋯⋯⋯⋯⋯⋯⋯⋯ 170

Siri ⋯⋯⋯⋯⋯⋯⋯⋯⋯⋯⋯⋯⋯ 109

six attributes of caring ⋯⋯⋯ 209

skiing ⋯⋯⋯⋯⋯⋯⋯⋯⋯⋯⋯ 40

sleep disturbance ⋯⋯⋯⋯⋯⋯ 52

society ⋯⋯⋯⋯⋯⋯⋯⋯⋯⋯⋯ 3

sociocultural perspective ⋯⋯⋯ 97

Stride Management Assist System

　(SMAS) ⋯⋯⋯⋯⋯⋯⋯⋯ 37, 38

stroke ⋯⋯⋯⋯⋯⋯⋯⋯⋯⋯⋯ 36

super-aged ⋯⋯⋯⋯⋯⋯⋯⋯⋯ 3

superintelligent machines ⋯⋯⋯ 214

surgical robots ⋯⋯⋯⋯⋯⋯⋯ 88

sympathetic relations ⋯⋯⋯⋯ 100

sympathy ⋯⋯⋯⋯ 87, 92, 100, 101

[T, t]

TAI ⋯⋯⋯⋯⋯⋯⋯⋯⋯⋯⋯⋯ 126

teachings of Buddha ⋯⋯⋯⋯ 124

Technological Competency as Caring in

　Nursing ⋯⋯⋯⋯⋯⋯ 176, 215, 217

technological

　— encounter ⋯⋯⋯⋯⋯⋯⋯ 215

— engagements ⋯⋯⋯⋯⋯⋯ 177

— knowing ⋯⋯⋯⋯ 212, 213, 216

— singularity ⋯⋯⋯⋯⋯⋯⋯ 232

technologies

　⋯⋯⋯⋯ 172, 210, 211, 213, 215-218

— (humanoid nurse robots) ⋯⋯ 210

tennis ⋯⋯⋯⋯⋯⋯⋯⋯⋯⋯⋯ 40

theoretical assumptions ⋯⋯⋯ 172

therapeutic relationship ⋯⋯⋯ 93

toileting aids ⋯⋯⋯⋯⋯⋯⋯⋯ 26

TON ⋯⋯⋯⋯⋯⋯⋯⋯⋯⋯⋯ 131

Transactive Relationship Theory of

　Nursing (TRETON) 168, 171, 215, 231

transactive relationships ⋯⋯ 168, 173

Travelbee's model ⋯⋯⋯⋯⋯ 227

tree structure system ⋯⋯⋯⋯ 100

trivialize activities ⋯⋯⋯⋯⋯ 149

trustworthy relationship ⋯⋯⋯ 87

Twitter ⋯⋯⋯⋯⋯⋯⋯⋯⋯⋯ 110

[U, u]

ultimate question ⋯⋯⋯⋯⋯⋯ 232

understanding ⋯⋯⋯⋯⋯⋯⋯ 89

Universal Technological Domain ⋯ 212

usefulness of ⋯⋯⋯⋯⋯⋯⋯⋯ 178

[W, w]

Walking Assist Robot ⋯⋯⋯⋯ 40

Index

WAR ································· 40, 43

Wearable Power-Assist Locomotor ·· 40

Wearable transfer aids ················ 21

Wearable type AI/Robot ·············· 129

WPAL ·································· 40, 41

Endorsements

I am Amazed at the Focus of This Work! Congrats! Jean

This remarkable book brings to the foreground the profound ethical and technological issues between technology of humanoid robots in Nursing and healthcare and human caring; it invites science fiction post human discourse and explorations for the future which is already before us. These authors are pioneering leaders in the field – bringing an entirely new world into our view for how we as humans sustain human caring in an emerging post-human era. A must-read text for faculty and students of Nursing and health sciences. For any thought leader in the industry!

Jean Watson, PhD, RN, AHN-BC, FAAN
Founder, Watson Caring Science Institute
Nursing theorist, Human Caring
www. Watsoncaringscience.org

Endorsements

Social Dilemma of Increasing Elder Care Needs in a World of Decreasing Younger Carer

This text bravely faces an ever emerging social dilemma of increasing elder care needs in a world of decreasing younger carer availability. While moral and ethical considerations are raised in the current and future use of robot technology, the authors scientifically present valid arguments for use of tireless technology in caring for humans, especially those with dementia, victims of stroke, and other chronic conditions. This book also celebrates and acknowledges the value of nurses transferring as many human caring realities to humanoid nursing robots as humanly possible, while maintaining oversight of caring science principles in the application of automated caring technologies.

Patrick J. Dean, RN; EDD, OSTJ
Clinical Associate Professor and Coordinator
University of Minnesota School of Nursing
International Association for Human Caring
President

Healthcare Tasks and Nursing Care Revisited

I believe the robots will have "healthcare tasks" delegated to them by nurses. In the United States of America (USA) nurses do not delegate nursing care, they delegate "healthcare tasks". In the US nursing care is protected and the knowledgeable assessments performed by registered nurses cannot be delegated. This is a really important issue. You may have something similar in Japan. YOU need to establish the role of nursing and helper robots and bring these forward to the Global Market – understanding the capacity of robots to assist nurses with healthcare tasks. I would be VERY happy to continue to assist with this great advancement.

Charlotte D. Barry, PhD, RN; NCSN, FAAN
Professor and Master Teacher
Florida Atlantic University
Christine E. Lynn College of Nursing
777 Glades Road

Biosketch of Authors

Barnard, Alan .... Chapter XIV

RN; BA, MA, PhD, is a faculty member of the School of Nursing at Queensland University of Technology (QUT) in Australia. He has a long-term interest in the philosophy of technology and nursing, as well as patient-focused care in both hospital and community environments. He is a Member of the QUT Institute for Health and Biomedical Innovation, and is an Honorary Research Fellow at a major teaching hospital in Australia. Dr. Barnard has received numerous awards, major research funding, and has in excess of seventy publications in international peer-reviewed journals and books.

Fuji, Shoko .... Chapter IV

RN; PHN, PhD is the deputy head nurse at the Sanaikai Mifune Hospital. She earned her BSN, MSN, and PhD from the University of Tokushima in 2011, 2013, and in 2016, respectively. Her research focuses on caring in nursing for older adults with dementia; especially for improving their autonomic nervous activity and activity in daily living.

Ito, Hirokazu .... Editor, Preface, Chapter XIII

RN; PhD earned his BSN, MSN, and PhD from the University of Tokushima in 2007, 2013, and 2016, respectively. He worked as a staff nurse at the Tokushima University Hospital in Japan from 2007 to 2013. He has been an Assistant Professor since 2013. His research focus is on improving the quality of nursing care. He developed the Psychiatric Nursing Assessment Classification System (PsyNACS©), a patient database in psychiatric nursing. Also, he focuses on ethical dilemmas in human caring involving human-humanoid robot interactions in nursing.

Kai, Yoshihiro .... Chapter V

Dr. Eng., is Professor of Robotics at the Department of Mechanical Engineering in Tokai University, Japan. He received his Bachelor's Master's degree, and his Doctor of Engineering degree in Mechanical Engineering from Doshisha University. From 1999 to 2002, he was a research associate at the Kochi University of Technology, Japan. Since 2003, he has been with Tokai University. His current research interests focus on the development of human-friendly

Biosketch

robots such as walking support robots for elderly people, exoskeleton robots, and service robots which support human daily activities.

Kato, Kaori .... Chapter IV
RN; BSN is a graduate student of nursing at the Tokushima University Graduate School of Health Sciences in Tokushima, Japan. She received the degree of Bachelor in Integrated Arts and Sciences from Hiroshima University in Hiroshima, Japan, in 1998, and the degree of Bachelor in Nursing Science from Tokushima University in Tokushima, Japan, in 2015. Her research interest is patient-family-centered care, and research focuses on technological competency as caring in nursing as perceived and their practicality for nurses in the Intensive/Acute Care Unit.

Koyama, Soichiro .... Chapter II
RPT, PhD is an assistant professor of the Faculty of Rehabilitation at the School of Health Sciences of Fujita Health University in Aichi, Japan. He earned his Doctor of Science from SOKENDAI (The Graduate University for Advanced Studies). His research focuses on neurophysiology, motor learning, brain stimulation, and developing activity-assist robots.

Locsin, Rozzano C. .... Editor, Prologue, Chapter X, XII, XIII, X IV, Epilogue
RN; PhD, FAAN is Professor of Nursing at the Tokushima University in Japan, Professor Emeritus at the Florida Atlantic University, and Visiting Professor at colleges of nursing in Thailand, Uganda, and the Philippines. He is the author of the volume Technological Competency as Caring in Nursing, which was translated into Japanese in 2015, and then revised in 2016. He is a nationally and internationally published author, an editor/co-author of three other books, a multi-awarded nurse scholar and educator, a Fulbright Scholar to Uganda, a Fulbright Senior Specialist in Global/Public Health and International Development, a member of the Philippine-American Academy of Science and Engineering (PAASE), and a Fellow of the American Academy of Nursing (FAAN).

Matsumoto, Kazuyuki .... Chapter VII
PhD is an assistant professor at the Graduate School of Tokushima University in Tokushima, Japan. He earned his PhD from Tokushima University. His research focuses on information

Biosketch

science, natural language processing, and affective computing. He is a member of the Information Processing Society of Japan (JSPI); the Association for Natural Language Processing (ANLP); and the Institute of Electronics, Information, and Communication Engineers (IEICE).

Omori, Mitsuko .... Chapter I
RN; BA, MA, MSN, PhD is a professor of geriatric nursing in the faculty of Medicine of Kagawa University in Kagawa, Japan. She earned her BA and MA from the Shikoku Gakuin University; she earned her MSN from Saint Luke's College of Nursing, Graduate School of Nursing Science, and finally her PhD from the Kawasaki University of Medical Welfare. Her research focuses on caring in nursing for older adults with dementia and the lived experience of terminally ill patients. She has translated into Japanese Dr. Rozzano C. Locsin's book Technological Competency as Caring in Nursing.

Orand, Abbas .... Chapter III
PhD is an assistant professor in the Rehabilitation Division of the Fujita Memorial Nanakuri Institute at the Fujita Health University in Tsu, Japan. He earned his PhD in the field of informatics and biosciences from Keio University. He obtained his MS in Mechatronics from Siegen University and his Bachelor of Electrical Engineering from Dalhousie University. His research focus is on healthcare technologies, robotics, wearable devices, human gaits, exoskeletons, and signal processing.

Osaka, Kyoko .... Editor, Preface, Chapter VI, XIII
RN; PHN, PhD, is a Lecturer of Nursing at the Graduate School of Tokushima University in Tokushima, Japan. She earned her PhD degree from Tokushima University. She has worked at Tokushima University since 2013. Her research interests are caring for the elderly with dementia, elderly and caring robot interaction, and empathic understanding in nursing.

Ren, Fuji .... Chapter VIII
Received his Ph. D. degree in 1991 from the Faculty of Engineering of Hokkaido University in Sapporo, Japan. Since 2001, he has been a Professor of the Faculty of Engineering of Tokushima University. He has been the president of the AIA International Advanced

256

Information Institute since 2003. His current research interests include Natural Language Processing, Artificial Intelligence, Affective Computing, and Emotional Robots. He is a senior member of IEEE, a member of AAMT, IPSJ, IEICE, CAAI, IEEJ; the Editor-in-Chief of International Journal of Advanced Intelligence, a vice president of CAAI, and a Fellow of The Japan Federation of Engineering Societies.

Sugawara, Kenichi .... Chapter II
RPT, PhD is the chief professor of the Physical Therapy Division at the Department of Rehabilitation of the Faculty of Health and Social Services at Kanagawa University Human Services in Yokosuka, Japan. He earned his PhD from Hiroshima University. His research focuses on neurophysiology, motor learning, motor control of motor cortex, and spinal motoneuron for paretic or normal limbs in rehabilitation situations.

Sugimoto, Hiroko .... Chapter IV
RN; PHN, BSN, MSN is a PhD student at the Graduate School of Health Sciences in Tokushima University, Japan. She earned her BSN and MSN degrees from Tokushima University. She is working as a nursing teacher at the elementary and junior high school in Tokushima, Japan. Her research interests in her PhD course are the relationship among mental and physical health, as well as among lifestyle, autonomic nervous activity, and the sleeping-waking rhythm in healthy people.

Takeda, Kotaro .... Chapter III
PhD is an associate professor in the Division of Rehabilitation at the Fujita Memorial Nanakuri Institute at the Fujita Health University in Tsu, Mie, Japan. He graduated from the Faculty of Science and Technology at Keio University in 2000. In 2007, he received his PhD in Science in Health Sciences from the International University of Health and Welfare. His research focuses on neuroscience, neurophysiology, ergonomic technology, and mechanical engineering; which includes robotics in rehabilitation. He is the Deputy Chief Editor of the Journal of Rehabilitation Neurosciences, Japan.

Biosketch

Tanabe, Shigeo .... Chapter II, III
RPT, PhD is an associate professor of the Graduate School of Health Sciences and of the
Faculty of Rehabilitation at the School of Health Sciences of Fujita Health University in Aichi,
Japan. He earned his BA and MS in rehabilitation (physical therapy) from Kawasaki
University of Medical Welfare, and his PhD in engineering from Keio University. His research
focuses on developing activity-assist robots to support caregiver (care assist), patient
(independence assist), and therapist (exercise assist).

Tanioka, Tetsuya .... Editor, Prologue, Chapter XI, XII, XIII, XIV, Epilogue
RN; PhD, FAAN is professor of nursing in the Department of Nursing Outcome Management
at the Tokushima University Graduate School in Tokushima, Japan. He earned his PhD from
the Kochi University of Technology. His research focuses on healthcare technologies, the
integration of science and technology within caring science, and robotics in nursing. He
received patents for his quintessential research on the PSYCHOMS ® system, or Psychiatric
Outcome Management Systems. He has translated into Japanese two state-of-the-art books on
caring: Boykin and Schoenhofer's Nursing as Caring, and Locsin's Technological
Competency as Caring in Nursing. He is Fellow of the American Academy of Nursing
(FAAN).

Yamazaki, Kazunori .... Chapter III
PhD is an assistant professor at the Faculty of Clinical Engineering in the School of Health
Sciences at the Fujita Health University in Aichi, Japan. He earned his Doctor of Engineering
degree from the Nagoya Institute of Technology in 2014. He is promoting development of
electronic devices and software aimed at improving the Quality of life (QOL) of human beings,
using a collaboration between medicine and engineering. His areas of expertise are medical
engineering, instrumentation technology, quantitative evaluation, proprioception, and
sensorimotor integration function.

Yasuhara, Yuko .... Editor, Preface, Chapter IV, XIII
RN; PHN, PhD, is an associate professor of nursing at the Department of Nursing Outcome
Management of the Tokushima University Graduate School in Japan. She received her MSN
from the Kobe City College of Nursing in 2003, and her PhD from the Kawasaki University of

258

Medical Welfare in 2013. She worked as a stuff nurse at hospital in Kobe, Japan from 1993 to 2000. She has worked at the Tokushima University since 2001. Her research focuses on sleep and the activity of people, care for patients with ischemic heart disease, safe intramuscular injection techniques, and caring as nursing.

Zhao, Yueren .... Chapter IX
MD; PhD, is a Lecturer at the Department of Psychiatry of the Fujita Health University in Aichi, Japan. He obtained his Doctor of Philosophy degree in 2013 from Kumamoto University. He started his carrier as an anesthesiologist in 1994, and bridged to psychiatry in 1997. He continues to work as a clinical psychiatrist, focusing on promoting good patient-physician relationship through open patient-oriented dialogue among multidisciplinary team members using approaches which strengthen anti-stigma activities. Dr. Zhao is a former board member of the Japan Young Psychiatrists Organization.
(JYPO; http://www.jypo.org/en/)

Foreword:
Savina Schoenhofer, RN, PhD

Endorsement:
Jean Watson, PhD, RN, AHN-BC, FAAN Founder Watson Caring Science Institute
Patrick J. Dean, RN; EDD, OSTJ
Charlotte D. Barry, PhD, RN; NCSN, FAAN

Editorial Assistants: Ms. Eri Umehara, Ms. Ryoko Bando
English Editor: Mr. Michael Gomez
Illustration/ Graphic Creator: Mr. Leo Vicente Bollos

JCOPY 〈(社)出版者著作権管理機構 委託出版物〉

本書の無断複写（電子化を含む）は著作権法上での例外を除き禁じられています。本書をコピーされる場合は、そのつど事前に(社)出版者著作権管理機構（電話 03-3513-6969、FAX 03-3513-6979、e-mail: info@jcopy.or.jp）の許諾を得てください。

また本書を代行業者等の第三者に依頼してスキャンやデジタル化することは、たとえ個人や家庭内での利用であっても著作権法上認められておりません。

Nursing Robots
Robotic Technology and Human Caring for the Elderly

2017 年 3 月 25 日　初版発行

編　著　者	谷岡 哲也，安原 由子，大坂 京子 飯藤 大和，Rozzano C. Locsin

発　　　行　**ふくろう出版**
〒700-0035　岡山市北区高柳西町 1-23
友野印刷ビル
TEL：086-255-2181
FAX：086-255-6324
http://www.296.jp
e-mail：info@296.jp
振替　01310-8-95147

印刷・製本　友野印刷株式会社
ISBN978-4-86186-689-0 C3047　Ⓒ2017

定価はカバーに表示してあります。乱丁・落丁はお取り替えいたします。

カバーデザイン、文中イラスト　ⒸLeo Vicente Bollos, 2017